Exceptional Bodies
in Early Modern Culture

Exceptional Bodies in Early Modern Culture

Concepts of Monstrosity before the Advent of the Normal

Edited by
Maja Bondestam

Routledge
Taylor & Francis Group
LONDON AND NEW YORK

The editors would like to thank the Swedish Research Council and the Ragnhild Blomqvist Foundation for their generous funding of the international workshop *Extraordinary bodies in early modern nature and culture,* that took place in Uppsala, Sweden, in October 2017 and from which several contributions to this book originated. The workshop was organized by the research programme *Medicine at the borders of life: Fetal research and the emergence of ethical controversy in Sweden* (medicalborders.se), supported by the Swedish Research Council (Dnr 2014–1749) and hosted by the Department of History of Science and Ideas at Uppsala University, Sweden.

First published in 2020 by Amsterdam University Press Ltd.

Published 2025 by Routledge
4 Park Square, Milton Park, Abingdon, Oxon OX14 4RN
605 Third Avenue, New York, NY 10158

Routledge is an imprint of the Taylor & Francis Group, an informa business

ISBN: 9789463721745 (hbk)
ISBN: 9781041179023 (pbk)
ISBN: 9781003695103 (ebk)
NUR 685

Cover illustration: Detail of the fetus in Johann Remmelin, 'First Vision', 1619. Etching and engraving from *Catoptrum microcosmicum*. Wellcome Library, London. Photograph: Rosemary Moore.

Cover design: Coördesign, Leiden

DOI 10.5117/9789463721745

For Product Safety Concerns and Information please contact our EU representative:
GPSR@taylorandfrancis.com
Taylor & Francis Verlag GmbH, Kaufingerstraße 24, 80331 München, Germany

The monster is by definition the exception.

– Michel Foucault, *Abnormal: Lectures at the Collège de France, 1974-1975*

Table of Contents

List of Illustrations

List of Illustrations

Introduction

Maja Bondestam

When a German scholar, Johan Jennings, sent a three-legged dove to the Swedish naturalist Carl Linnaeus in 1748, the response was lukewarm. Linnaeus thanked Jennings officially for the gift in the proceedings of the Royal Swedish Academy of Science and incorporated the bird in the society's collection of natural objects. In a letter to another colleague, however, Linnaeus stated that society not should publish an article about the find, since readers would only be bored with another malformation. According to Linnaeus, three-legged birds appeared every year, were not rare anymore and piqued the interest of naturalists only when anatomized professionally.[1] Naturalists around Europe collected and exchanged odd and unexpected minerals, plants and animals by this time, and Linnaeus's actions reveal how the value of such bodies increased in relation to their rareness. Nothing was exceptional in itself, and the impression a three-legged dove would make depended on its audiences and on their expectations and experiences of the world. The perception of something as exceptional, rare and valuable – or not – depended on a person's identity, prior knowledge and sense of what strayed from the ordinary path of things.[2]

Historians today have come to similar conclusions and connected exceptional bodies to the examination of monsters, monstrosity, disability, defects and wonders. Cultural historian Surekha Davies describes 'monster studies' as the study of that which appears strange to our eyes.

> In the broadest sense, monsters are beings that fall outside the viewer's ontological categories in some way; a two-headed calf and a new animal species both constitute monsters in this sense. Monsters, and our own puzzlement about them, are thus entry-points to a deeper understanding of a culture's way of thinking.[3]

1 Linné, *Bref och skrifvelser*, pp. 120-121.
2 Garland, *The Eye of the Beholder*, pp. 5-7.
3 Davies, *Renaissance Ethnography*, p. 14.

Bondestam, M. (ed.), *Exceptional Bodies in Early Modern Culture: Concepts of Monstrosity before the Advent of the Normal.* Taylor & Francis Group, 2020
DOI 10.5117/9789463721745_INTRO

To define a monster, its impact and effects must be examined, Asa Simon Mittman argues in his introduction to a volume on the subject.[4] In a similar way, historians of disability have paid attention to the observer, more than the observed. 'I define physical disability as a disruption in the sensory field of the observer', writes Lennard J. Davis.[5] Lorraine Daston and Katharine Park claim in their seminal *Wonders and the Order of Nature, 1150-1750*, that wonders generally had to be 'rare, mysterious and real not to be dismissed as common deviances' and that they, together with monsters, made up a long-lived cluster of strange objects and phenomena.[6]

The three-legged dove perhaps did not puzzle or disturb Jennings and Linnaeus in their ontological categories, but it definitely had some impact on them and might have disrupted their sensory fields. The dove was real for both of them; it was rare for Jennings but not for Linnaeus, who is famous for his all-embracing and systematic ordering of nature into species and subspecies, classes and families, but also for wondering about curious naturalia and the amazing diversity of creation.[7] According to Linnaeus, the collecting of engraved wood blocks, fossils, bones, optical instruments, coins, bezoars, so-called unicorn horns, corals, birds of paradise and elaborate works in gold, silver and ivory was time well spent. He saw natural explanations as evidence of God's existence and believed for this reason that unexpected, strange and peculiar animals, plants and minerals had the power to move people deeply. Such bodies were supposed to direct the observer's thoughts towards important narratives of the origin of nature and to make the audience understand its own origin and duties better than before.[8]

In his dismissal of the three-legged dove, Linnaeus appears in the traditional guise of the natural philosopher, a 'man who, by debunking their rarity and elucidating their causes, was able to make wonders cease'.[9] Wonders, monsters, and prodigies, however, did not cease that easily. They populated the early modern world; were displayed, collected and described; and reminded people of unpredictable, new and diverse possibilities. A dove with three legs was an exception from the common rule, exempt from the ordinary, well-known and conventional order of things.

The chapters in this book deal with bodies outside all conventions around Europe in the sixteenth, seventeenth, and early eighteenth centuries. Taken

4 Mittman, 'Introduction', p. x.
5 Davis, 'Dr. Johnson', p. 56.
6 Daston and Park, *Wonders*, pp. 10, 17.
7 Broberg, *Mannen som ordnade naturen*, pp. 139-150, 284-286, 313-337.
8 Linné, 'Naturens ordning', p. 63.
9 Daston and Park, *Wonders*, p. 165.

together, seven case studies reveal a variety of approaches to exceptional bodies before the advent of a modern norm, which in the seventeenth century started to represent all deviances as close and relative to a homogenous standard. The bodies in focus were in their own historical contexts sometimes called monstrous, prodigious or hermaphroditic, and to our late modern eyes they can appear as disabled, unruly, transboundary, dying or deviating from some prescribed position. The volume includes bodies of stillbirths, monsters of maternal imagination, exalted experiences of prodigious births, hermaphrodites as figures of theological inquiry, the effect of physical aberrations on social standing and career, the use of the rhetoric of monstrosity to regulate women's sexuality and moderations of the exercising body. It explores concepts of monstrosity in an expanding early modern Europe and examines how cultural representations and policies incorporated physical deviances before the advent of modernity and its emerging universal standard for the normal body, with its emphasis on health and beauty.

As the case studies will show, exceptional bodies functioned as ways to understand and order the world. They could convert into hierarchies and identities and denote the limits of nature, power, legitimacy, virtue, history, and the human body. In terms of monsters and monstrosity, they actualized connections between specific bodies and an all-embracing cosmic order but could also be ignored and dismissed as irrelevant errors. Before the emergence of a modern, standardized and hegemonic norm centred on the contours of an adult, able-bodied, European man, exceptional bodies could be frightening, good, bad, worth considering, irrelevant, curious and part of people's way of understanding the origin of nature and humanity. Monstrous, prodigious and hermaphroditic bodies framed the porousness of living beings, informed concepts of life and death, the strange and odd. They displayed expected power relations, a certain gender order, hierarchies between humans and animals and the boundaries of a moderate way of life. In this volume, we want to deepen the historical understanding of this range of meanings and propose a narrative based in historically specific tendencies, competing perspectives and local truths. Rare and truly exceptional bodies are at the centre of attention, as are their dynamic meanings, complex social relations and power relations in specific circumstances. To study the function of monsters and monstrosity in the early modern period, as previous research has shown, can help us gain greater understanding of the culture that produced them.[10] The contributors to this volume analyse

10 Deutsch and Nussbaum, *'Defects'*; Mittman, 'Introduction', p. 9.

experiences, meanings, metaphors and the use and value of exceptional bodies in a period when, according to Michel Foucault, it was monstrous bodies, not behaviours, that evoked the most serious response.[11]

We move from France, the Dutch Republic and Rome to Germany, Sweden and the globally expanding Spanish Empire in the search for a broad spectrum of experiences, and examine a variety of source materials. The volume brings together exceptional bodies from the middle of the sixteenth century to the early eighteenth century and focuses on medicine and natural philosophy but also on early modern culture in a more inclusive sense. Visual culture, satirical poems, novels, political treatises, mirrors for princes, plays, theological inquires, philosophy, court medicine, anatomical flap books, dictionaries, birth manuals, autobiographies and written collections of wonders and monsters are analysed as sites for establishing social relations and order. The transgressive field of monster studies can contribute to our knowledge of physical rules and exceptions, although the object of study is notoriously difficult to define. Where do we look if we are interested in monstrosities, and how do we know that we have found them? What was the nature of monstrous existence before the middle of the eighteenth century? Was a disabled body a monster? What do we call a body with so many different layers of meaning?

The remainder of this introduction suggests some answers to these questions. It relates the volume at hand to earlier research on disability, monsters and wonders as a way to circumscribe the exceptional body in the early modern period. As mentioned already, the case studies examine specific bodies in specific cultural and historical contexts. Here we call them *exceptional* because they could be both outstanding and extraordinary in a positive way and, in a more negative sense, deviations from the general picture, ugly, disturbing, frightening or simply irrelevant. Jennings and Linnaeus acted in relation to this tension in the middle of the eighteenth century, but as we will see, it has a longer history.

Early modern bodies and the advent of the normal

Scholars often say that it is productive to study monsters and deviances, defects, deformities and disabilities because they reveal what a society considers as normal when it comes to physical appearance and competence. Historian David M. Turner underscores that the ways in which 'a society

11 Foucault, *Abnormal*, pp. 67-75.

defines disability and whom it identifies as deformed or disabled reveal much about that society's attitudes and values concerning the body, what stigmatizes it, and what it considers "normal"'.[12] This is true in modernity but not as much for the early modern period. In this book, we deal with the value of rare, wondrous, boundary-breaking, frightening and odd corporeality in a range of cultural environments and in a period when a modern Western framework did not define physical deviances in relation to an average standard or statistical norm. We see the early modern period neither as one in which monsters emerged as 'crucial definitional Others in the process of European self and nation formation' nor as a time 'when the modern self – self-determining, individual, self-knowing' – was being created.[13] Monsters before 1750 often had to do with visual difference and exceptions from expected shapes or identities. We cannot, however, take for granted that they always contributed to cultural dichotomies or binary oppositions such as beautiful and ugly, perfect and grotesque, self and Other, subject and object, or that they participated in the mutual constitution of the desired norm and the deviant Other.

The presence of monstrous Others, so often referred to in the field of monster studies, can be questioned before the late eighteenth century. At least if we assume that people did not yet see nature as an absolutely regular and universally homogenous entity, compared natural variations on a common scale, or related exceptional bodies to statistical norms and average standards.[14] Pliny's monstrous races and their afterlife in the first period of colonization were definitely part of early modern culture as they showed up in maps of non-European parts of the world. Nevertheless, it is not certain that they related to the Europeans in the same way before, as after, the late eighteenth century.

Helen Deutsch and Felicity Nussbaum claim that when attempts in the eighteenth century were made to define difference as a natural fact, and not as a sign of divine or preternatural agency, the monster was revealed 'as the norm's inverse reflection'.[15] This sentence is interesting in two ways. First, it suggests that the norm has a history, which seems reasonable.

12 Turner, 'Introduction', p. 2. See also Gilbert, Wiseman and Fudge, *At the Borders of the Human*, p. 8. Jeffery Jerome Cohen argues that the monster is best understood as 'an embodiment of difference, a breaker of category, and a resistant Other known only through process and movement, never through dissection-table analysis'. Cohen, 'Preface', p. x.

13 Knoppers and Landes, 'Introduction', p. 7.

14 Said, *Orientalism*, pp. 21-24, 116-121, 126-127, 149-141; Fabian, *Time and the Other*, pp. 106-107, 143; Foucault, *The Order of Things*, p. 155.

15 Deutsch and Nussbaum, *'Defects'*, p. 13.

Second, it suggests that monsters have been seen as natural facts only since the eighteenth century, which is harder to agree with. Already in medieval natural philosophy, monsters were, as Daston and Park have shown, explained by natural causes and only seldom by the involvement of divine or demonic powers.This was still the case during most part of the seventeenth century, even while omens were being taken seriously in European elite culture. Monsters were not *naturalized* before 1750, they were *normalized*, which was a slow process, characterized by multiple explanations and uneven courses of events.[16]

The norm has a history, and so does its relation to physical deviances, which some scholars encourage us to take seriously. Lennard J. Davis emphasizes that the norm is more the effect of a certain kind of society than a universal condition of human nature. He connects it with notions of nationality, race, gender, criminality and sexual orientation, which emanated from the late eighteenth century onwards. 'The word "normal" as "constituting, conforming to, not deviating or differing from, the common type or standard, regular, usual" only enters the English language around 1840.'[17] The concept emerged in European culture through statistics and political arithmetic, medicine and public health. The Belgian statistician Adolphe Quetelet combined *l'homme moyen physique* and *l'homme moyen morale* and in 1835 constructed both a physical and moral human average. The average man was the man in the middle, celebrating moderation and the middle way of life; according to Davis, the bourgeois hegemony had its scientific legitimation in this figure. The average was paradoxically associated with greatness, beauty and goodness and the concept of the norm invited the majority of the population to be part of or to relate itself to the norm. Davis contrasts this to earlier societies and encourages us to see a situation when the hegemony of normalcy did not exist. He describes a premodern era and the relevance of a mytho-poetic, ideal body, the nude Venus or Helen of Troy, linked to the gods and to a divine and ideal body which was not attainable by humans, since an ideal never could be found in this world. Classical painting and sculpture idealized the body, smoothing out every particularity, whereas all members of the population were below the ideal and never expected to conform to it.[18]

In the volume at hand, we are interested in early modern monstrosity and examine exceptional bodies in relation to their historical specific

16 Daston and Park, *Wonders*, p. 14, 129, 176, 192-193, 205.

17 Davis, *Enforcing Normalcy*, p. 24.

18 Ibid., pp. 24-27, 29.

contexts. This means that we do not see them as smaller versions of modern ones, as the norm's inverse reflection, or as entangled with a culture in which binary concepts of the normal and the abnormal, the self and the Other, were fundamental. As discussed by Jennifer Terry and Jacqueline Urla, such dynamics of difference, constructions of bodies and dependent relationships appeared in the nineteenth century, when the normal body as an unmarked figure started to gain its meaning 'mainly in residual contrast to various deviant bodies'.[19] Modern vernaculars of rationality, hygiene and bureaucratic order made the sorting of different peoples an imperative and 'fuelled a feverish desire to classify forms of deviance, to locate them in biology, and thus to police them in the larger social body'.[20] This ordering of differences, bodies, identities and power relations was part of heated debates about legal end economic privileges, who they were and were not for, in the modern democracies from the late eighteenth century onwards.[21]

In the 1970s, Foucault discussed eighteenth-century processes of individualization and normalization, which involved meticulous observation and examination of differences between individuals. With reference to Georges Canguilhem's book *On the Normal and the Pathological*, he described a general process of social, political and technical normalization during the eighteenth century that became important in the domains of education, medicine, hospital organization and industrial production. The century saw the invention of new technologies of power, which are important in relation to medicine and physical deviances today. 'We pass from a technology of power that drives out, excludes, banishes, marginalizes, and represses, to a fundamentally positive power that fashions, observes, knows, and multiplies itself on the basis of its own effects.'[22] The word 'positive' may indicate that the new technologies were a good thing but what Foucault identified was rather a shaping and modifying power in modernity. Based on the norm, this power brought with it a principle of both qualification and correction. 'The norm's function is not to exclude and reject. Rather, it is always linked to a positive technique of intervention and transformation, to a sort of normative project.'[23] In processes of normalization, individuals were established, fixed, given presence and a place of their own but also exposed for 'constant examination

19 Terry and Urla, 'Introduction', pp. 4-5.
20 Ibid., p. 1.
21 Garland-Thomson, *Extraordinary Bodies*, pp. 63-70; Laqueur, *Making Sex*, chap. 5; Scott, 'Some More Reflections', pp. 201-202, 214-218; Wahrman, *The Making of the Modern Self*, pp. 83-87, 92-93, 113-117, 127-129, 143, 152-153.
22 Foucault, *Abnormal*, p. 48.
23 Ibid., p. 50; Canguilhem, *The Normal*, pp. 125-149.

of a field of regularity within which each individual is constantly assessed in order to determine whether he conforms to the rule, to the defined norm of health'.[24] This is something other than marginalizing, distancing, ignoring, killing or placing monsters as far away as possible.

In their edited volume on monsters in early modern Europe, Laura Lunger Knoppers and Joan B. Landes point to the same passages in Foucault's lectures and state that monsters, like the category *early modern*, 'blur boundaries as well, transgressing, violating, polluting, and mixing what ought to be kept apart'.[25] They search for links between the monstrous and the political and read representations of monsters in relation not only to science but also to religious and political conflict, transformations in print and the rise of the nation-state. Knoppers and Landes study the monstrous on a metaphorical level: its polemic, literary and imaginative uses. How did the language of the monstrous work, what was the significance of monstrous bodies, what emotional responses did they call up and how did myths of monstrosity figure in understandings of self and Other?[26]

In the volume at hand, we follow up on such questions before the advent of a modern physical norm. We are not saying that bodies in the sixteenth, seventeenth, and early eighteenth centuries lacked order and boundaries, or were without prescriptions and prohibitions, but that rules and exceptions from rules were something other than what they are in modernity.[27] In the early modern period there were often clear definitions of what made a proper body and explicit rules for marriage, sexual relationships and inheritance in relation to people's physical capacities. Linnaeus, for example, was impressed by the number of well-behaved (*artiga*) animals, plants and minerals in creation and by appropriate kinds and species whose characteristics followed general habits and established customs.[28] His world was so full of exemplary naturalia that he could not bother to keep track of the erroneous ones as well. He said this in a time when all creation was understood to be pervaded by God's benevolent intentions and inclinations, in which people found values

24 Foucault, *Abnormal*, p. 47.

25 Knoppers and Landes, 'Introduction', p. 6.

26 Ibid., pp. 14-15.

27 Rules underwent, according to Lorraine Daston, a noteworthy change in the eighteenth century and moved from the rule-as-model to the rule-as-algorithm. Whereas most rules of the sixteenth and seventeenth centuries were elastic, leaving room for judgement and adjustment, using examples as well as appeals to experience and even to exceptions, the regulations of the eighteenth century became increasingly rigid in their formulation. Daston, *Rules*.

28 Linnaeus, *Bref och skrifvelser*, p. 71. On the habits of early modern nature, see Daston and Park, *Wonders*, p. 14; Park, 'Nature in Person', pp. 53, 56, 60, 64, 73.

and guidelines, indications of what was right and wrong. Early modern nature had a certain moral authority and functioned as a source for moral judgements and considerations.[29] According to Daston and Park, morality joined with nature in prearranged harmony, which charged aberrations with meaning, 'whether as warnings from an angry God, sports of playful nature, or blemishes in the uniformity of the universe'.[30]

Elements, humours and complexions built up early modern bodies and connected them with wider environments, with nature, climates and geographies, and a search for similarities and analogies was a fundamental part of how single bodies echoed macrocosmic orders.[31] There were in the early modern era judicial restrictions on marriage and employment for infertile persons, and we can study disabilities, physical irregularities and stigmas to grasp their meanings and aims as well as important categories and values of their societies. Monsters, hermaphrodites, prodigies and all kinds of strange, frightening, erroneous, ominous, transgressing and wondrous bodies and phenomena populated the early modern world. They disturbed legislation, classification of species, rules of physical heritage and concepts of time, and existed as categories of their own. Monsters undermined definitions, challenged boundaries, made people think differently and were genuinely difficult to sort. They sometimes indicated the presence of higher orders and were, through a symbolic system, connected with cosmos as a whole.[32]

To say that early modern monsters reveal a related *norm* can be misleading. Rules before the eighteenth century were often elastic; nature had room for exceptions, and the social order for judgement and adjustment, whereas deviances were not necessarily the opposite of what was right or desirable. Exceptional bodies could also arouse wonder and remind people of a playful nature and of God's freedom and power. Early modern nature had moral authority, bodies were idealized and particularities were evened out. In line with historian Dror Wahrman I would say that identities before the middle of the eighteenth century were generic and had room for deviances and that they not yet were objects of curable operations, of comparisons on a common scale or of examinations in relation to some average body in the statistical middle.[33]

29 Daston and Vidal, 'Necessity and Freedom', p. 206.

30 Daston and Park, *Wonders*, p. 363.

31 Davies, *Renaissance Ethnography*, pp. 25-26; Groebner, '*Complexio*/Complexion'; Deutsch and Nussbaum, '*Defects*', p. 9; Hanafi, *The Monster*, pp. 100-120.

32 Eriksson, *Monstret & människan*, pp. 39-45, 268-269, 278, 280, 309, 322-323.

33 Daston, 'The Nature of Nature', p. 154; Wahrman, *The Making of the Modern Self*, pp. 182-185, 276-278.

Early modern monstrosities are an exciting field of research because they unveil concepts of corporeality in a period when people in their daily lives often followed other rules and rationalities than those we have become used to. They deviated from a nature that was ordered by habits, purposes and higher reasons; they were charged with meaning; and their history differs from other periods. One aspect of early modern monstrosity is that exceptional bodies not only were considered degrading and dehumanizing but also evoked curiosity and intellectual interest. This alertness to historical peculiarities is central in this volume.

The nature, location and significance of the monster

The word *monster* has multilayered meanings. The Latin *monere* means 'to warn, remind and encourage'; *monstrum* refers to that which is worthy of warning, reminding, or encouraging; whereas *monstrare* means 'to show or demonstrate'.[34] In the ancient world, a *monster* was something outside the existing order of nature. Aristotle considered anomalous births as monsters and defects of nature. Anything that did not resemble its parents, particularly its father, was a monster in his view. Even women, who lacked the perfection of men, were a kind of monster. The Aristotelian monster did not illustrate or portend anything. It was not ominous, shocking or frightening and had no divine or demonic connections.[35]

Cicero defined monsters as portents of the will of the gods, whereas Saint Augustine, in line with the teratological tradition represented by Pliny the Elder, considered both monstrous births and the legendary races of the East to show God's power and remind men that no law of nature circumscribed him. Monsters could remind men of the limitations of their knowledge, according to Augustine. It was not that these creatures were monstrous; it was that man was not capable of understanding the sense and order of God's diverse creation. God was here an omnipotent artist who repeatedly awoke a sense of wonder.[36]

A tradition, important from the Middle Ages onwards, associated monsters with manifestations of God's will and displeasure. They aroused dislike, fear, repugnance, and were associated with bad omens but also with amusement, fun, gifts from God and physical challenges.[37] John Block Friedman describes

34 Knoppers and Landes, 'Introduction', p. 3.

35 Davies, 'The Unlucky', p. 50.

36 Eriksson, *Monstret & människan*, pp. 128-132; Hanafi, *The Monster*, pp. 7-14.

37 Godden and Mittman, *Monstrosity*, pp. 4-5.

a strong interest in divination and prodigies in Renaissance thought as well, and claims that monstrous forms fascinated and terrified because they challenged peoples understanding of the human and reminded people of the uncertainty of traditional concepts of man.[38]

An interest in strange bodies connects to the use of striking and thought-provoking examples in early modern culture, and so does the activity of collecting exceptional bodies and things. Natural philosophers, physicians and collectors of naturalia and curiosities in the fifteenth and sixteenth centuries were not preoccupied with revealing false wonders, omens and monsters. Instead, as Paula Findlen and Camilla Mordhorst have shown, they used monstrosities to understand nature, explain the inexplicable and find recurring principles in an irregular world.[39] Findlen reads the collecting of rare naturalia in relation to the empirical explosion of materials by this time, the spreading of ancient texts, increased travel, voyages of discovery and new forms of communication and exchange.[40]

The outstanding capacity of monsters to surprise, to arouse admiration and wonder, was part of their value as a path to homiletic knowledge and enhanced virtue. Krzysztof Pomian notes that viewers of wondrous bodies would ideally remember something specific in the creation or in social life and be encouraged to act in a certain way. In European elite culture, at the courts, and in trade, travel and among collectors of naturalia this approach embraced everything exceptional, odd and rare. Cabinets of curiosity or *Kunst- und Wunderkammern* were, in the sixteenth and seventeenth centuries, part of a tradition that highly valued noteworthy and extraordinary objects and bodies. Paradoxically, the collecting of rarities could in time lead to questions concerning their rarity and exceptional nature. The great number of extraordinary naturalia showed when they gradually appeared in large series, weaving them into larger patterns of systematicity, continuity, kinship and regularity in nature. Natural philosophers compared objects in the same homogenous class and let them explain each other.[41] Jennings's wish to collect odd animals and Linnaeus's more blasé attitude have already given us a glimpse of this devaluation of natural collections in the middle of the eighteenth century.

A lot is known about the changing nature, location and significance of monsters also when we narrow the time period to the sixteenth, seventeenth and

38 Friedman, *The Monstrous Races*, pp. 3, 108-130.

39 Findlen, *Possessing Nature*, pp. 1-3, 71; Mordhorst, *Genstandsfortællinger*, p. 184.

40 Findlen, *Possessing Nature*, p. 3.

41 Pomian, *Collectors and Curiosities*, pp. 64, 91-92.

early eighteenth centuries and before I define the subject of this book more precisely, a handful of the most often referred scholars will be introduced.

According to historian Michael Hagner, there were monsters everywhere in seventeenth-century Europe. They appeared as subjects for conversation, in discussions and anecdotes, and functioned as curiosities and entertainment at courts and markets. Learned journals represented monsters as case studies, and for natural philosophers and collectors they were desired objects to put in cabinets. Monsters did not generate feelings of fear or superstition but of wonder, at least at courts and universities, and Hagner examines how that changed during the Enlightenment. Significant shifts had to do with the understanding of life as a *process* in the eighteenth century, with the rise of a more regular and predictable order in nature, a new focus on beauty and with an intensified classification of deviances and differences in science. Hagner calls the monster a revealer of power in the so-called Age of Reason and suggests that universal laws and deterministic processes were overshadowing the old playful, artistic nature by the beginning of the eighteenth century. An effect was that monsters no longer were seen as unusual, wonderful and curious.[42]

A focus on power is central also in Foucault's monster studies. He claimed that, from the Middle Ages to the eighteenth century, the *monster* was essentially a mixture of two realms, kingdoms or species, such as the animal and the human. It could also be a blending of two individuals, the two sexes or of life and death, such as when a child was born with some morphology that meant it would die in hours or in a few days. The child was not able to live but survived nonetheless for a short period, which made it monstrous. The monster could finally be a mixture of forms, and a person who, like a snake, had no arms or legs, was a monster. Monsters transgressed natural limits and classifications, but the breach of natural law was not enough to constitute monstrosity in seventeenth- and eighteenth-century thought.[43] A monster also had to disturb some interdiction of civil or religious law, and the difference between disability and monstrosity revealed this.

> Disability may well be something that upsets the natural order, but disability is not monstrosity because it has a place in civil or canon law. The disabled person may not conform to nature, but the law in some way provides for him. Monstrosity, however, is the kind of natural irregularity that calls law into question and disables it.[44]

42 Hagner, 'Enlightened Monsters', pp. 175-178.
43 Foucault, *Abnormal*, pp. 63-64.
44 Ibid., p. 64.

It was, according to Foucault, only when the confusion of a mixed body also overturned or disturbed civil or canon law and created disorder in social life that it became a question of monstrosity. Should shapeless infants inherit from their parents? Was it reasonable to baptize an offspring with two heads once or twice? Was it possible to sentence a conjoined twin to death, or did the authorities then also kill an innocent person? Could a hermaphrodite marry, and with whom?[45] Monstrosity was fundamentally a *juridical-natural* concept, troubling both natural boundaries and the law.

Closer to our own time, Foucault described *the abnormal individual*, an everyday monster, or *the individual to be corrected*. This figure appears clearly in the eighteenth century, can be seen already in the seventeenth century, but much later than the monster, whose frame of reference was nature and society, the system of the laws of the world. The individual to be corrected had a narrower frame of reference and emerged in the play of relations of conflict and support that existed between the family and the school, workshop, street, quarter, parish, church, police and so on. This figure became much more frequent than the monster ever was and it was typically regular, so to speak, in its irregularity. The individual to be corrected always appeared close to the rule, familiar, difficult to define, exhibiting a number of ambiguities that we will encounter again, long after the eighteenth century, in the problematic of the abnormal man. 'The monster is by definition the exception; the individual to be corrected is an everyday phenomenon.[46]

Does this mean that we find *monsters* in the early modern era and *individuals to be corrected* from the eighteenth century onwards? Nothing is easy in the history of monstrosities, and scholars in the field seldom agree. One narrative is that physically extraordinary persons before the end of the seventeenth century could have a prominent place in culture, carry meaning and remind people of God's presence. They had a playful nature, could be displayed, display themselves, travel and arouse wonder and excitement. During the eighteenth century, all kinds of extraordinary bodies were transformed into mute deformations, distanced from anything elite, simply vulgar. Monsters were embedded in the context of embryology and comparative anatomists extended their knowledge of the normal organism by placing it in relation to these anomalies. Monsters disappeared from streets and marketplaces at the same time as they entered scientific tables and examination rooms, and this once-challenging, original, wondrous,

45 Ibid., pp. 63-64.
46 Ibid., p. 58.

rare and sometimes threatening category was approved of to the extent that it disappeared.[47]

There are, however, disruptions, and overlapping tendencies in this trajectory and Stephen Pender underlines continuity. He reminds us that the reception of the monster as full of meaning did not simply expire at a certain point, nor was there a principal line of development from monsters as prodigies to monsters as medical pathologies. His research on conjoined twins in the seventeenth century reveals a more fluid interchange between the portentous and the merely anomalous. Pender claims that monsters' political and theological resonance remained important and demonstrates how monsters continued to occasion emblematic thought in cabinets, at birth scenes and at exhibitions throughout the century.[48]

If monsters were rare but seen and displayed on many cultural levels in the early modern period, it seems to have been the opposite with disabilities. Davis describes an absence of discourse on the topic before 1750. He sees the term *disability* as tied to the emergence of discourses that 'aim to cure, remediate, or catalogue variations in bodies' and claims that researchers have had difficulty finding disability before the middle of the century.[49] This is not because variations in ability did not exist, but because disability was not yet an operative category. Physical differences were not pathologized and Davis discusses the historical and cultural transition in which the modern discourse of disability became consolidated. Whereas people with disabilities did not receive much attention, there was in the seventeenth and early eighteenth centuries an inordinate amount of interest in wonders, *lusus naturae*, giants, dwarfs, hermaphrodites, conjoined twins, hirsute women and anomalous births. Today we would perhaps define such conditions as disabilities, but the grouping together of birth anomalies and disability did not exist much before the nineteenth century.

> Our modern concept of normality requires that all deviations from the norm be treated equally, but under the previous discursive grid, anomalous, strange births were distinguished from disabilities that were acquired, particularly through disease.[50]

47 Garland-Thomson, *Extraordinary Bodies*, pp. 70-80; Daston and Park, *Wonders*, pp. 18-20, 204-205; Park and Daston, 'Unnatural Conceptions', pp. 51-54; Canguilhem, *The Normal*, pp. 125-149; Hagner, 'Vom Naturalienkabinett', pp. 73-78; Hagner, 'Enlightened Monsters', p. 178; Curran, 'Afterword', pp. 230-231.

48 Pender, '"No Monsters"', pp. 147, 162.

49 Davis, *Enforcing Normalcy*, p. 56.

50 Ibid., p. 59.

Davis observes a new discursive category of disability from the middle of the eighteenth century, along with 'the development of an institutional, medicalized apparatus to house, segregate, isolate, or fix people with disabilities'.[51] A medical gaze took the place of staring at wonders, and Davis claims that disabled persons now became observed, commented on, illustrated, treated, dissected, legally placed and inscribed into an economy of bodily traits. In addition, mental illnesses were categorized in types and subtypes, and the concept of normality was invented along with bell curves and statistics.[52]

In this volume, we approach exceptional bodies and concepts of monstrosity before the advent of such a norm. We focus on dramatic instances of physical deviance, monsters, prodigious births and hermaphrodites but also on metaphorical monstrosities and on bodies with the power to disrupt the sensory field of the observer. Our monsters are exceptions rather than individuals to be corrected, and precise analyses of how monstrosity worked in specific contexts are made throughout the book. It is far from surprising that we are more generous in the demarcation of the research object than Foucault, who claimed that monstrosity disrupts both natural and judicial laws. Our topic is also wider than that described by Asa Simon Mittman, who defines monsters and the monstrous as 'threats to common knowledge' that cast doubt on people's 'epistemological worldview'.[53] The exceptional bodies we meet in the volume at hand could definitely act as threats or shape new worldviews, but not only this. They were often rare, unruly, disruptive or wondrous but could also be ignored and dismissed, as exemplified by Linnaeus. Exceptional bodies both astonished and bored people in the early modern period, and this paradox is present in a number of the case studies. The boring side of monsters can be traced back to Aristotle and the scholastics, described briefly below, before the individual case studies in this volume are introduced.

The epistemology of the monstrous: Practices, knowledge, morals, affect

Disregard for monstrosities was an important part of learned culture long before the eighteenth century. Aristotle saw monsters as errors of nature, not

51 Ibid., p. 61.
52 Ibid., p. 62. See also Garland-Thomson, *Extraordinary Bodies*, pp. 63-70; Foucault, *The Birth of the Clinic*, pp. 89-90, 100, 105, 107-108, 112-121.
53 Mittman, quoting Noël Coward, in 'Introduction', p. 8.

portending anything, and his medieval followers rejected irregular bodies as inappropriate for natural philosophers to examine since they deviated from the general picture. The nature of the accidental is the topic here; a temporary, particular, random and failed by-product, which was irrelevant for or even contradicted the essential body in which it appeared. Scholastic natural philosophy marginalized wonders and monsters in the search for regularity in nature, and this attitude persisted throughout the thirteenth and fourteenth centuries.[54]

Philosophers who aspired to *scientia*, defined by Aristotle as 'certain knowledge', should produce not only probable or possible facts but universally true 'science'. This rigorous epistemological ideal was not easy to apply in relation to the shifting and irregular physical world, as opposed to the unchanging nature of God, and one strategy became to study *types of phenomena* and *universal principles* rather than *particularities*. Bodies and events beyond the ordinary course of nature, such as conjoined twins, rains of blood, monstrous births or individual prodigies, were ignored and seen as the result of unspecifiable causes that were combined in unforeseeable ways. Resulting in singular and utterly contingent bodies, such combinations and processes were, in scholastic natural philosophy, seen as outside the realm of the necessary and universal.[55]

Chapter 5 in this volume connects with the Aristotelian tradition in early modern culture to value universal types more highly than actual bodies and specific cases. Here, Parker Cotton examines how the French philosopher Pierre Bayle, in the interesting and complex web of articles and cross-references comprised in his *Dictionnaire historique et critique* (1697), located the hermaphrodite in mythology rather than in his own time and reality. The individual case, the local and particular hermaphrodite with a certain shape, character and rootedness in time and space, was not as interesting as the original man, a mythic category, an ideal and a generic type before the Fall. Ovid's Salmacis, the hermaphroditic first man; Adam in Eden; or a monster on a distant continent fuelled Bayle's discussion on hermaphrodites and filled the contours of an exemplary and historical figure with power to change contemporary understandings of divine creation or to give the reader a lesson. The whole issue reveals the persistence of repulsion towards actual and singular bodies even in late-seventeenth-century philosophy and an emerging intellectual discussion about the first man, which made it possible for Bayle to challenge a dogmatic and rigid theology

54 Daston and Park, *Wonders*, pp. 110-112, 120, 126.

55 Ibid., pp. 114-117.

of his time. 'I believe Bayle's repeated connections of hermaphroditic figures to mythic origin stories offer an ongoing challenge, or reappraisal, of the original state of humanity,' writes Cotton.

The exceptional body also has a more positive conceptual history, far from the Aristotelian generic type, which connects it with the playful and wondrous dimensions of nature, its freedom to deviate from rules and the ability to awake wonder and reveal aspects of human origins and the world's creation. Daston and Park have contributed in many ways to our understanding of monsters, hermaphrodites and wonders before 1750. They show, for example, how the category of wonders embraced a crowd of strange objects and phenomena, such as expensive and unusual animals, plants and naturalia as well as courtly spectacles of various kinds. In the fifteenth and sixteenth centuries, wonders offered pleasure and delight, were seen as sports of a creative and variable nature, as exotic, representing wealth and power, and were valued for their sophistication, strangeness and refinement. Monsters belonged intermittently to this category, and people showed them to each other because of their novelty and capacity to surprise and astonish.[56] Exceptional bodies and things became desirable to own, brought both knowledge of the physical world and the reputation that all men of learning cultivated.[57]

The desire for exceptional bodies as wonders can also be found in various court practices, where, in the same way as a piece of clothing and a rare, exotic or luxurious object, they transcended prosaic experience and contributed to a specific aesthetics. In Chapter 1, Maria Kavvadia analyses the tensions surrounding dance culture in sixteenth-century Rome. Religious and medical discourses overlapped in the work of Girolamo Mercuriale, court physician of one of the most powerful cardinals in Rome in the middle of the century, and Kavvadia lets us follow his regulation of a certain dance, the *moresca*. She shows us that in relation to the Counter-Reformation and the Catholic Church, there was a cultural circulation of medical, moral and religious rules and orders and a search for ancient origins, which emphasized the value of moderation, health and order. Mercuriale was not satisfied with how the *moresca* was performed in his own time and promoted 'ancient dance culture [...] as an example, a model to be followed', as Kavvadia remarks.

A discontentedness with exceptional bodies within the interpreter's own cultural context, accompanied by a fascination with ancient ones, appears

56 Ibid., pp. 101-103, 190-191, 193-201.

57 Findlen, *Possessing Nature*, p. 3.

not only in the writings of Bayle and Mercuriale but throughout the early modern period, and so does the tension between particular bodies and the study of generic types. This changed, however, during the early modern period and monster studies is a good place to start for anyone interested in the shifting value of particular bodies in relation to universal categories and types. Case studies and actual bodies, monstrous, prodigious and hermaphroditic ones as well, were represented in sixteenth- and seventeenth-century medicine, in collections of wonders and curiosities and in learned elite culture. Individual lives and deaths appeared in obstetrics, so did personal witnessing and the practical aspects of extraordinary births.[58]

The presence and value of monsters and wonders in the seventeenth century is complex, and at the end of the century the questions of what a prodigious birth was and what one should do with it were still far from resolved. Living beings were expected to produce offspring resembling themselves, and during this century there was a persisting correspondence between microcosm and macrocosm, between the human body and God's wider creation. 'Man is a little world, made in the image of God', as Zakiya Hanafi reminds us.[59] Imitation and similitude were central concepts in seventeenth-century medicine, so what should be done with children missing essential organs, with two heads instead of one or exhibiting hairy instead of naked skin? Chapter 6 in this volume contains my discussion of the so-called prodigious son of a fisherman, born on the east coast of Sweden in the 1660s, and deepens these questions. I analyse the ways in which the humanist and professor of rhetoric and government Johannes Schefferus recalled the most noteworthy things he had come across during his life. In 1668 he described, in his handwritten 'Variae historiae', monstrous births as well as kidney stones, poisonous mines, memorable stories and archaeological findings, and this collection of wondrous and memorable things and bodies makes the case that exceptional bodies should be displayed to people to improve their virtue and knowledge.

Here we are far from the scholastic tradition in which natural philosophers avoided monsters and exceptional bodies as accidental and irrelevant errors in nature, and closer to the tradition of *exempla*, in which fictive and real persons' lives and actions, as well as exceptional bodies and monsters, were represented as models for people to follow or avoid. This tradition relates to the notion of history, nature and culture as being filled

58 Ibid., pp. 1-5; Pomian, *Collectors and Curiosities*, pp. 64, 90-92; Bates, *Emblematic Monsters*, p. 57; Davies, 'The Unlucky', p. 75.

59 Hanafi, *The Monster*, p. 102.

with homiletic and edificatory examples, mirroring timeless knowledge and providing a path for acquiring virtue. In the sixteenth century, there emerged a whole genre of popular prodigy tales, reprinted and augmented well into the seventeenth century. One constantly expanding volume was *Histoires prodigieuses*, in which different authors during the second half of the century produced one book after the other on both ancient and contemporary wonders. Pierre Boaistuau wrote the first one and gave the volume its title in 1560.[60]

Both *looking* at exceptional bodies and *collecting* them in cabinets and books could be a good thing but what about the physical processes that *produced* them? Rosemary Moore argues in Chapter 2 that maternal imagination and visual imprinting were not only perilous, corrupting, dangerous and unruly aspects of the female anatomy but also part of a productive nature, giving rise to new life forms. Women's gazing on images of perfect male babies could have a positive impact on their fetuses and work as a way to control and positively influence the outcomes of their pregnancies. Moore takes the slippery and ambiguous nature of maternal imagination as an alternative theoretical framework for understanding the conflation of allegorical, religious and medical imagery in the early seventeenth century. In analyses of 'fugitive sheets', anatomical broadsheets whose cut and layered structures carry multiple meanings and ambivalences, she replaces rigid dichotomies and sees, both in pregnant bodies and in medical prints, a lack of stability and an openness to interpretation. A sophisticated reading of the materiality, spatiality and interactive dimensions of anatomical flap books connects us in this chapter with multifaceted, printed layers of the body, carefully arranged to mimic spatiality, specific organs and allegorical symbols. Moore focuses on the 'First Vision' from the physician Johann Remmelin's *Catoptrum microcosmicum* (Mirrors of the microcosm) triptych of fugitive sheets, published in 1619, and shows us that the monster or Medusa's head, which intriguingly forms part of it, was associated with knowledge, virtue and an active nature. 'I hope that this might begin to open up a dialogue about the multiplicities of meanings that can be found just below the surface of Remmelin's print, and of its many possible uses, misuses and (mis)interpretations at the hands of different users,' writes Moore.

Chapter 3 deals with the close relation between body and soul, as well, and with physical and moral beauty. Pablo García Piñar analyses bodily deviance in a globally and administratively expanding seventeenth-century Spanish Empire and focuses on the Mexican playwright and lawyer Juan

60 Eriksson, *Monstret & människan*, pp. 133-136; Daston and Park, *Wonders*, pp. 180-189.

Ruiz de Alarcón's path to public office. García Piñar examines the language of perception, beauty, perfection, bodily malformation and disability in political treaties, mirrors for princes, satirical poems and pieces, novels and plays from the 1620s and discusses the correspondence between Ruiz de Alarcón's body and the morals of colonial administration. Visual impressions and mediations in satires and plays functioned, along with general notions of the body, as legitimizing sources of authority, and García Piñar analyses the tension between the manner in which a body was formed and the expected behaviour and capabilities of the person. By following a playwright and his fictional characters, García Piñar works at the intersection of early modern literature and disability studies and grasps the experience of being marginalized. 'Don Juan represents the first case – and perhaps the only one – of an early modern disabled character conceived by an author with a disability, that is, created from the embodied experience of being in a disabling world,' he writes.

Exceptional bodies both challenged and supported the ordering of the early modern social world, and so did monstrous sexuality when displayed and demonstrated for larger audiences. Through an analysis of the satirical piece *Divorce satyrique* (1660), which stages the fake confession of Henri IV, king of France, Cécile Tresfels, in Chapter 4, examines representations of feminine power and the sexuality of the king's ex-wife, Marguerite de Valois. In this specific context, the negative function of monstrosity was used on a symbolic level, and the purpose of the satire was to debase the king via the alleged monstrosity of his wife's sexuality. Tresfels shows us a complex set of cultural, political and emotional features, mechanisms and consequences of the satire. The narrator in *Divorce satyrique* underlines that Marguerite's monstrosity comes from within and that her extraordinary sexuality is driven by internal desire. 'Her deformed body is a consequence and manifestation of this internal monstrosity, reflecting materially the depravity of her soul.' In line with Foucault, one could say that Marguerite was an individual to be corrected, a pale monster with too much power, exhibiting behaviour in supposed need of intervention. She was not a monster in the *juridical-natural* sense, a natural transgression or troubling of the law, and it should be noticed that Tresfels' case call into question Foucault's timeline and his clear distinction between early modern and modern practices.

We obviously need to know more about how physical, sexual and behavioural exceptions were conceptualized in the early modern period. How did ideal types, *exempla* and virtue work together and were modern *norms* something entirely different? Daston and Park emphasize the emergence of strict norms and absolute regularity, both of nature's customs and God's rules, from the late seventeenth century onwards. Nature's habits hardened into inviolable laws, and new attitudes towards nature were established among natural philosophers who faced 'the subordination of anomalies to watertight natural laws, of nature to God, and of citizens and Christians to established authority'.[61] The natural order became uniform, lost room for exceptions, and in an eighteenth-century anatomical framework monsters were transformed into organisms that failed to achieve their perfect final form. They were normalized and placed in relation to a functional standard and their value now depended, not on their rarity or singularity, as in earlier times, but on the body's capacity to reveal still more encompassing and rigid regularities. The history of monsters as submitted to these strict norms, rather than to secular powers, can be traced for many decades and seen still in the early nineteenth century. Daston and Park close their *Wonders and the Order of Nature* in 1750 and state that monsters were by then reduced to an incomplete part of nature, which in itself became uniform across time and place. There was no enlightenment, disenchantment or clear pattern of naturalization taking monsters from prodigies, by way of wonders, to naturalistic objects.[62]

Daston and Park are convincing in their argument that wonders and monsters not were naturalized or secularized in the seventeenth century, as well as in their description of rare and extraordinary wonders being reduced to distasteful errors in the early eighteenth century. They spend, however, fewer words on the actual process of normalization. What was it, how was it expressed, and where do we find it?

In the volume at hand, we examine exceptional bodies and monstrosity before the emergence of a modern, statistical norm and average standard. We approach early modern sources and try to be sensitive about their historically specific orders and disorders, rules and exceptions, on the level of the body. In Chapter 7 Tove Paulsson Holmberg examines perinatal children as liminal beings. She focuses on stillbirth in late-seventeenth- and early-eighteenth-century Sweden, tracing the ambiguous, conditional character of unborn corporeality in case studies of emergency obstetric practices. The chapter is about suffering and death in the birth transition, which for centuries had been an expected part of labour, positioning the survival of the mother against the survival of the child. With the pioneering Swedish gynaecologist Johan von Hoorn, who around 1700 introduced

61 Daston and Park, *Wonders*, p. 208.

62 Ibid., pp. 176, 187, 189, 192-193, 202, 205-209, 214, 329, 361.

active obstetric methods, the conditions changed to some extent. New examination and intervention techniques demarcating and describing obstructed, 'unnaturally' positioned unborn babies made these marginal entities visible, yet, in the beginning of the eighteenth century, the manifest presence of perinatal loss continuously framed all medical and religious practices related to the birth transition. Modern obstetrics would eventually change the expectations of life and death, which again reminds us that the value and meaning of the exceptional body is relative to its viewers and to its cultural and historical contexts.

Taken together, some key themes recur in these chapters. One is the relation between monstrous behaviours and monstrous bodies, and another is how extraordinary bodies have functioned as a path to knowledge and virtue. Throughout the book, we analyse the unstable boundaries between exceptional bodies and their audiences, as well as rules and expectations in relation to physical deviances. Monstrosity, hermaphroditism and prodigious births function as a way to create order, authority, and political and emotional stability. In a concluding afterword, Kathleen Long reflects upon these themes, on the value of exceptional bodies and on the concepts of monsters and monstrosity before the advent of the normal.

Through seven essays, chronologically organized, this volume makes the claim that exceptional bodies not only challenged social, religious, sexual and natural structures and hierarchies in sixteenth-, seventeenth- and early-eighteenth-century Europe but also contributed to its knowledge, moral values and emotional repertoire. The case studies show that monsters and monstrosity were part of a heterogeneous material world in which they evoked forgotten categories, remarkable creations and memorable rarities. At the same time, exceptional bodies, sometimes in the terms of monstrosity, had a function in relation to political reasoning, created order, delivered critique and enhanced certain messages. Prodigious births, maternal imagination, collections of extraordinary experiences and things, hermaphrodites, powerful women, bodily deviances, ambiguous stillbirths, controversial moves and exercises, shapeshifting phenomena, and hybrids of various kinds were part of an ongoing categorization and ordering of bodies, behaviours, social relations and hierarchies. In a period when customs rather than strict norms were supposed to dominate the processes of nature, monstrosities could contribute to human experience in the most unexpected and sometimes positive ways. Odd, rare, original and unique bodies, practices and phenomena were in certain circumstances not that bad, wrong and frightening after all.

Works Cited

Bates, A.W., *Emblematic Monsters: Unnatural Conceptions and Deformed Births in Early Modern Europe* (Amsterdam: Rodopi, 2005).

Broberg, Gunnar, *Mannen som ordnade naturen. En biografi över Carl von Linné* (Stockholm: Natur & Kultur, 2019).

Canguilhem, Georges, *The Normal and the Pathological*, with an introduction by Michel Foucault, trans. Carolyn R. Fawcett in collaboration with Robert S. Cohen (New York: Zone Books, 1989).

Cohen, Jeffery Jerome, 'Preface: In a Time of Monsters', in *Monster Theory: Reading Culture*, ed. Jeffery Jerome Cohen (Minneapolis: University of Minnesota Press, 1996), pp. vii-xiv.

Curran, Andrew, 'Afterword: Anatomical Readings in the Early Modern Era', in *Monstrous Bodies/Political Monstrosities in Early Modern Europe*, ed. Laura Lunger Knoppers and Joan B. Landes (Ithaca: Cornell University Press, 2004), pp. 227-245.

Daston, Lorraine, 'The Nature of Nature in Early Modern Europe', *Configurations* 6, no. 2 (1998), pp. 149-172.

Daston, Lorraine, *Rules: A Short History of What We Live By* (Princeton: Princeton University Press, forthcoming).

Daston, Lorraine, and Ferdinand Vidal, 'Necessity and Freedom', in *The Moral Authority of Nature*, ed. Lorraine Daston and Ferdinand Vidal (Chicago: University of Chicago Press, 2004), pp. 205-206.

Daston, Lorraine, and Katharine Park, *Wonders and the Order of Nature, 1150-1750* (New York: Zone Books, 1998).

Davies, Surekha, *Renaissance Ethnography and the Invention of the Human: New Worlds, Maps and Monsters* (Cambridge: Cambridge University Press, 2016).

Davies, Surekha, 'The Unlucky, the Bad and the Ugly: Categories of Monstrosity from the Renaissance to the Enlightenment', in *The Ashgate Research Companion to Monsters and the Monstrous*, ed. Asa Simon Mittman with Peter J. Dendle (Abingdon: Routledge, 2012), pp. 49-75.

Davis, Lennard J., 'Dr. Johnson, Amelia, and the Discourse of Disability in the Eighteenth Century', in *'Defects': Engendering the Modern Body*, ed. Helen Deutsch and Felicity Nussbaum (Ann Arbor: University of Michigan Press, 2000), pp. 95-126.

Davis, Lennard J., *Enforcing Normalcy: Disability, Deafness, and the Body* (London: Verso, 1995).

Deutsch, Helen, and Felicity A. Nussbaum, eds, *'Defects': Engendering the Modern Body* (Ann Arbor: University of Michigan Press, 2000).

Eriksson, Jonnie, *Monstret & människan: Paré, Deleuze och teratologiska traditioner i fransk filosofi, från renässanshumanism till posthumanism* (Lund: Sekel bokförlag, 2010).

Fabian, Johannes, *Time and the Other: How Anthropology Made Its Object* (New York: Columbia University Press, 1983).

Findlen, Paula, *Possessing Nature: Museums, Collecting, and Scientific Culture in Early Modern Italy* (Berkeley: University of California Press, 1994).

Foucault, Michel, *Abnormal: Lectures at the Collège de France, 1974-1975*, ed. Valerio Marchetti and Antonella Salomoni; English series editor, Arnold I. Davidson; trans. Graham Burchell (London: Verso, 2003).

Foucault, Michel, *The Birth of the Clinic: An Archaeology of Medical Perception*, trans. A.M. Sheridan Smith (New York: Vintage Books, 1994).

Foucault, Michel, *The Order of Things: An Archeology of the Human Sciences* (New York: Vintage Books, 1994).

Friedman, John Block, *The Monstrous Races in Medieval Art and Thought* (Syracuse: Syracuse University Press, 2000).

Garland, Robert, *The Eye of the Beholder: Deformity and Disability in the Graeco-Roman World* (Ithaca: Cornell University Press, 1995).

Garland-Thomson, Rosemarie, *Extraordinary Bodies: Figuring Physical Disability in American Culture and Literature* (New York: Columbia University Press, 2017).

Gilbert, Ruth, Susan Wiseman and Erica Fudge, eds, *At the Borders of the Human: Beasts, Bodies and Natural Philosophy in the Early Modern Period* (Basingstoke: Macmillan, 1999).

Godden, Richard H., and Asa Simon Mittman, 'Embodied Difference: Monstrosity, Disability, and the Posthuman', in *Monstrosity, Disability, and the Posthuman in the Medieval and Early Modern World*, ed. Richard H. Godden and Asa Simon Mittman (Cham: Springer International, 2019), pp. 3-31.

Groebner, Valentin, '*Complexio*/Complexion: Categorizing Individual Natures, 1250-1600', in *The Moral Authority of Nature*, ed. Lorraine Daston and Ferdinand Vidal (Chicago: University of Chicago Press, 2004), pp. 361-383.

Hagner, Michael, 'Enlightened Monsters', in *The Sciences in Enlightened Europe*, ed. William Clark, Jan Golinski and Simon Schaffer (Chicago: University of Chicago Press, 1999), pp. 175-217.

Hagner, Michael, 'Vom Naturalienkabinett zur Embryologie: Wandlungen des Monströsen und die Ordnung des Lebens', in *Der Falsche Körper: Beiträge zu einer Geschichte der Monstrositäten*, ed. Michael Hagner, 2nd ed. (Göttingen: Wallstein, 2005), pp. 73-107.

Hanafi, Zakiya, *The Monster in the Machine: Magic, Medicine, and the Marvelous in the Time of the Scientific Revolution* (Durham: Duke University Press, 2000).

Knoppers, Laura Lunger, and Joan B. Landes, 'Introduction', in *Monstrous Bodies/ Political Monstrosities in Early Modern Europe*, ed. Laura Lunger Knoppers and Joan B. Landes (Ithaca: Cornell University Press, 2004), pp. 1-22.

Laqueur, Thomas, *Making Sex: Body and Gender from the Greeks to Freud* (Cambridge, MA: Harvard University Press, 1990).

Linné, Carl von, *Bref och skrifvelser af och till Carl von Linné, Afd. 1. D. 2 Skrifvelser och bref till K. Svenska vetenskaps-akademien och dess sekreterare* (Stockholm: Ljus, 1908).

Linné, Carl von, 'Naturens ordning', in *Om undran inför naturen och andra latinska skrifter* (Stockholm: Natur & Kultur, 2005), pp. 61-109.

Mittman, Asa Simon, 'Introduction: The Impact of Monsters and Monster Studies', in *The Ashgate Research Companion to Monsters and the Monstrous*, ed. Asa Simon Mittman with Peter J. Dendle (Abingdon: Routledge, 2012), pp. 1-14.

Mordhorst, Camilla, *Genstandsfortællinger: Fra Museum Wormianum til de moderne museer* (København: Museum Tusculanums Forlag, 2009).

Park, Katharine, 'Nature in Person: Medieval and Renaissance Allegories and Emblems', in *The Moral Authority of Nature*, ed. Lorraine Daston and Ferdinand Vidal (Chicago: University of Chicago Press, 2004), pp. 50-73.

Park, Katharine, and Lorraine J. Daston, 'Unnatural Conceptions: The Study of Monsters in Sixteenth- and Seventeenth-Century France and England', *Past and Present* 92, no. 1 (1981), pp. 20-54.

Pender, Stephen, '"No Monsters at the Resurrection": Inside Some Conjoined Twins', in *Monster Theory: Reading Culture*, ed. Jeffery Jerome Cohen (Minneapolis: University of Minnesota Press, 1996), pp. 143-167.

Pomian, Krzysztof, *Collectors and Curiosities: Paris and Venice, 1500-1800*, trans. Elizabeth Wiles-Portier (Cambridge: Polity Press, 1990).

Said, Edward W., *Orientalism* (London: Penguin, 2003).

Scott, Joan W., 'Some More Reflections on Gender and Politics', in *Gender and the Politics of History*, rev. ed. (New York: Columbia University Press, 1999), pp. 199-222.

Terry, Jennifer, and Jacqueline Urla, 'Introduction', in *Deviant Bodies: Critical Perspectives on Difference in Science and Popular Culture*, ed. Jennifer Terry and Jacqueline Urla (Bloomington: Indiana University Press, 1995), pp. 1-18.

Turner, David M., 'Introduction', in *Social Histories of Disability and Deformity* (London: Routledge, 2006), pp. 1-16.

Wahrman, Dror, *The Making of the Modern Self: Identity and Culture in the Eighteenth-Century England* (New Haven: Yale University Press, 2004).

About the Author

Maja Bondestam is Associate Professor in History of Science and Ideas at Uppsala University. She has published books and articles on themes including politics of the maturing body, the history of the Swedish hermaphrodite, botanical classification, the language of Carl Linnaeus and gendered norms in medical advice literature.

1. The *Moresca* Dance in Counter-Reformation Rome: Court Medicine and the Moderation of Exceptional Bodies

Maria Kavvadia

Abstract

In the early modern elite court culture, dance held a prominent socio-political position. Nevertheless, in the Counter-Reformation era, the Catholic Church put dance culture under scrutiny. The *moresca*, one of the most popular dance spectacles that expressed the elite's taste in exceptional and wondrous bodies, was criticized as deviant by Catholic reformers. In this criticism, the religious discourse often overlapped with contemporary medical discourse, which considered aspects of dance culture as unhealthy for both body and soul. In Counter-Reformation Rome, Girolamo Mercuriale, the court physician of Cardinal Alessandro Farnese, following the aspirations of the Counter-Reformation papacy for spiritual reform, moderates in his medical treatise *De arte gymnastica* the controversial *moresca*: by modifying it into a medical exercise, he regulates the *moresca* in both medical and religious terms, making it an appropriate body practice for the elite.

Keywords: court medicine, medical gymnastics, early modern antiquarianism, medical illustration, early modern body culture

Over the last decades, dance has developed into a major historical discourse and area of historical study; research has demonstrated the centrality of dance, its social, political, educational, medical, moral, ethical and aesthetic resonances in early modern culture and society.[1] In social and

1 On sixteenth-century dance culture, see the work of Julia Sutton, Margaret McGowan and Jennifer Nevile. For the role of dance in early modern medicine as well as medical, moral and

Bondestam, M. (ed.), *Exceptional Bodies in Early Modern Culture: Concepts of Monstrosity before the Advent of the Normal*. Taylor & Francis Group, 2020
DOI 10.5117/9789463721745_CH01

anthropological studies dance has been described as a cultural practice and social ritual that functions as a means of aesthetic pleasure and a means for establishing ties and structure in a community.[2] Dance has also been described as a specific language that constitutes a social-historical phenomenon that depends on the space and time in which it exists and on the ruling power structures.[3]

Considering the above and in the framework of the volume at hand, the present essay looks into dance culture in the context of court medicine in Counter-Reformation Rome, teasing out sixteenth-century notions of exceptional and wondrous bodies, concepts of bodily order, disorder and deviance, as well as practices of moderation and regulation of exceptional bodies. The broad spectrum of the society's preoccupation with dance in the early modern period is demonstrated in the vast publication of dance literature (and literature for dance music) as well as in the numerous theological, medical and legal discourses that showed significant attention to dance and reveal to us the vigorous debates on its nature and moral value. Foucault's notion of discourse as articulated in his *Archaeology of Knowledge*[4] is enlightening in the framework of the present volume; in scholarly studies of extraordinary, exceptional and monstrous bodies 'the discourse in which a conversation is embedded will not only influence the vocabulary of the discussion but also have a large influence on the conclusions drawn', Richard Godden writes.[5]

The question on the nature and moral status of dance was not a new one in the early modern world; it went back to early and classical Christian texts that criticized dancing as lascivious and pagan. However, it was in the era of the Reformation and Counter-Reformation that the issue acquired particular prominence. Religious sources, both protestant and Catholic, displayed strong opposition to dancing, arguing that it was inappropriate for a pious Christian.[6] In a time when, after the Council of Trent,[7] the political-religious authorities of Rome put body culture under scrutiny, one of the dance genres

religious attitudes towards dance in the Counter-Reformation era, see the work of Alessandro Arcangeli.

2 Pušnik, 'Introduction', p. 5; see Radcliffe-Brown and Evans-Pritchard, *Structure and Function*.

3 Pušnik, 'Introduction', p. 5; see Bourdieu, *Language*.

4 Foucault, *Archaeology of Knowledge*.

5 Godden, 'Embodied Difference', p. 20.

6 Arcangeli, 'Dance under Trial', p. 127.

7 The Council of Trent was held between 1545 and 1563 in the city of Trent (or Trento) in northern Italy, and it was the nineteenth ecumenical council of the Catholic Church. It was prompted by the Protestant Reformation and it has been described as the embodiment of the Counter-Reformation.

severely criticized by the protagonists of the Counter-Reformation was the *moresca*,[8] which was an important part of the elite culture and part of the elite's fascination for wonders and extraordinary corporeality. The present essay brings forward the medical discourse of the humanist physician Girolamo Mercuriale (1530-1606)[9] on the *moresca*. It looks into the medical treatise *De arte gymnastica* (Venice, 1569)[10] that Mercuriale put together during his residence in Rome (in the years 1562-1569), where he served as the court physician of Cardinal Alessandro Farnese (1520-1589), one of the most eminent and powerful churchmen and richest patrons at the time. In his *De arte gymnastica* Mercuriale promotes the Greco-Roman gymnastics (or art of exercise) as an ideal method of medical treatment with preventive and curative value, for both body and soul. Following the ancient medical authorities, he identifies dance as part of medical gymnastics and in this framework, he examines the *moresca* as a medical exercise.

The essay, taking into consideration the idiosyncrasies that stem from the Catholic Reformation, the dual nature of Rome and the worldly nature of its ecclesiastical courts, brings forward Mercuriale's medical discourse on the *moresca* as a historical example which, owing to the prominent position of the *moresca* in elite courtly lifestyle, reveals tensions and shifting attitudes towards exceptional bodies and body practices. Following Lorraine Daston's and Katharine Park's assumptions regarding the early modern court as a space for the historical study of the body and body culture,[11] the aim of this essay is to contribute to our knowledge of early modern exceptional and wondrous bodies by looking into ways that court medicine negotiated courtly body culture in the Counter-Reformation era. By focusing on the *moresca* as a cherished court spectacle of wondrous bodies, and the discourse of

8 *Moresca*, or *morisco*, or morris; *moresche* in plural. The *moresca* will be described in greater detail later in the essay.

9 On the life and work of Girolamo Mercuriale, see the editions of *De arte gymnastica* by Agasse, Galante, Napolitano and Pennuto, as well as Sutton, *Sixteenth Century Physician*.

10 The book was first published in Venice in 1569. The full title of the first edition of the book reads as follows: *Artis gymnasticae apud antiquos celeberrimae, nostris ignoratae, libri sex In quibus exercitationum omnium vetustarum genera, loca, modi, facultates et quicquid denique ad corporis humani exercitationes pertinet, diligenter explicatur. Opus non modo medicis, verum etiam omnibus antiquarum rerum cognoscendarum et valetudinis conservandae studiosis admondum utile. Auctore Hieronymo Mercuriali Foroliviensi Medico et Philosopho. Medico & Philosopho* (Venetiis [Venezia], Apud Iuntas, In officina Iuntarum, MDLXIX [1569]). The first edition of the book was dedicated to Cardinal Alessandro Farnese, Mercuriale's patron at the time. The present essay draws from the critical edition of Girolamo Mercuriale's *De arte gymnastica* edited by Concetta Pennuto and translated into English by Vivian Nutton, henceforward cited as DAG.

11 Daston and Park, *Wonders*, pp. 100-108.

Mercuriale, as the court physician of one of the most eminent cardinals of the time, this essay aims: 1) to demonstrate the tensions between elite body culture and the religious-moral aspirations and demands of the Catholic Church, and 2) to throw light on the role of medicine in the process of regulating and moderating the exceptional body based on values shared by medical and religious authorities alike.

The first part of the essay highlights the manifold significance of dance for elite courtly culture. In this context, the second part introduces the *moresca* as a court spectacle of exceptional bodies and social identities. The next part discusses briefly the space of the elite courts in Counter-Reformation Rome, providing the background for a thick description[12] of Mercuriale's *De arte gymnastica* that brings forward his endeavour to moderate dance culture and the *moresca* according to a mixture or medical and moral-religious criteria.

A public spectacle of wonder and representation of power

Throughout the sixteenth century, dance was everywhere: at elite courts, in town squares and marketplaces, in stately ballrooms as well as in rural villages. In theory and practice, and as a source of literary inspiration, dance was a major preoccupation.[13] Dance made part of the elite's leisure and public display etiquette. It had an omnipresent role in the life of the Italian elites and was of major significance in both private and state occasions. In large state spectacles, as well as in private celebrations, dance was an important element through which the status and the power of the elite were publicly consolidated, magnified and expressed to the rest of the society.[14] Jennifer Nevile describes dance as a significant tool in the representation of power and social rank through rituals and ceremonies.[15]

Exploring dance in the context of early modern courts can be particularly fruitful, not least for its nature as an extraordinary spectacle for audiences to wonder. According to Daston and Park, for each elite group, wonder bore different meanings and implications.[16] The court interest in wonders took many forms and served specific political, social and

12 See Geertz, 'Thick Description'.
13 McGowan, *Dance*, p. 248.
14 Nevile, *The Eloquent Body*, pp. 52-56.
15 Ibid., pp. 8-9.
16 Daston and Park, *Wonders*, pp. 14-18.

cultural aims responding to historical circumstances. For example, it was expressed through collections of members of the elite, which exhibited rare, unusual and luxurious objects that were meant to represent the wealth and power of the collector, offer pleasure and delight, and cause astonishment to the spectators. Overall, the early modern court notion of the extraordinary identified with the fascination of the elite with the exotic and the strange, usually of foreign origin. Whether this was an object, an animal, a product or a piece of clothing, it formed a specific aesthetic that embodied political and cultural realities, messages and aspirations responding to historical circumstances. Among the early modern court practices and spectacles that demonstrate the elite's taste in the extraordinary and reveal notions of exceptional, extraordinary bodies and body culture, we find the *moresca*.[17]

The moresca: Exhibiting the exceptional, manifesting identities

The *moresca* was a mixture of theatrical, pantomimic and social dancing,[18] frequently performed in elaborate stage shows during formal state occasions (e.g. banquets, jousts and tournaments, theatrical performances, etc.) by courtiers as well as 'professional' dancers. It was found throughout Europe from the thirteenth century onward, thus, as a dance genre it encompassed a wide variety of elements.[19] However, we can discern the general characteristics of the *moresca*, at least as far as the early modern Italian dance culture is concerned.

According to Barbara Sparti, *moresche* were

> performed, for the most part, in costume, they [*moresche*] made use of distinctive headgear, masks, scenery and special effects – fire in particular. They portrayed allegorical, heroic, exotic and pastoral scenes. Mock skirmishes were common, the Fool was a popular character and the grotesque was frequently represented by doddering old men and fantastic monsters.[20]

17 Ibid., p. 101.

18 For further discussion on the *moresca* and an interpretation of its features, see Nevile, *The Eloquent Body*, pp. 12-57; Locke, Music and the Exotic, pp. 17-125; Sparti, 'Dancing in Fifteenth-Century Italian Society', pp. 53-57; McGinnis, Moving in High Circles, pp. 171-176; Forrest, History of Morris Dancing, pp. 74-90; Sparti, 'The Function and Status of Dance', pp. 42-61.

19 Nevile, *The Eloquent Body*, p. 33; Arcangeli, 'Dancing Savages', p. 292.

20 Sparti, 'Dancing in Fifteenth-Century Italian Society', p. 54.

Moresche featured masks, elaborate, sumptuous costumes (made of precious fabrics) and headpieces, props, sets, themes or brief storylines, mime, dance, including expressive gestures and larger movements beyond the accepted range of the dignified courtier, though some danced well-disguised in these interludes.[21] *Moresche* also featured danced combat and other pantomimic dancing, including the depiction of agricultural work, exotic characters such as wild men, allegorical figures such as vices and virtues, and mythological figures such as Hercules and centaurs. The performers were often masked or had their faces and hands blackened; blackness contributed to the Renaissance sense of the 'exotic'.[22] Furthermore, *moresche* also depicted rural activities, particularly in the later fifteenth century when it became almost synonymous with the dance known as *intermedio*.[23]

Jennifer Nevile describes *moresche* as 'danced dramas' in the sense that in them the elite dramatically defined their civilized identity by showing scenes of both civilization and barbarism. The appearances of wild men, savages or barbarians in *moresche* were one way of declaring 'this is what we are not', Nevile writes.[24] For the spectators and participants at the festivals, the wild men would be 'exotic', that is, outlandish, barbarous, strange and uncouth.[25] Here, the blackened faces and hands of the *moresca* dancers could be seen as representing the barbarian, the person who exists outside the limits of society.[26]

As such, the well-established dance spectacle of the *moresca* constituted a manifestation of the elite's taste in the exceptional and wondrous bodies. However, at the same time, it appeared disturbing and deviant in the theological climate of the Counter-Reformation.

Roman courts, the Catholic Reformation and the need for moderation

In the political-religious environment of the Counter-Reformation, such dance spectacles conflicted with the ethic of the Catholic reformers, who sought austerity in conduct, manners and attitudes, decorum, gravity, self-control, diligence, order, prudence, reason, sobriety and thrift. It is important

21 Ibid., p. 53-57; Sparti, 'The Function and Status of Dance', p. 44-45.
22 Nevile, *The Eloquent Body*, p. 144.
23 Ibid., pp. 33-34.
24 Ibid., p. 141.
25 Ibid., p. 143.
26 Ibid., p. 47.

to consider that papal Rome was both a religious and political centre and that the Roman courts, although mostly ecclesiastical in number, were as worldly in their lifestyle as the lay elite courts. The cardinals' courts exhibited power, wealth, sumptuousness, luxury and, overall, their etiquette was very much assimilating lay princely courts. In fact, Mercuriale's patron, Cardinal Alessandro Farnese, was renowned for holding one of the most grandiose courts in Rome.[27] However, this worldliness was considered problematic in the Catholic Reformation; it was seen as one of the vulnerabilities of the Roman Catholic Church for which Rome was severely attacked by protestants.[28] Hence, the members of the ecclesiastical elite were forbidden to participate in occasions that involved dancing and they were expected to conduct with decorum and gravity appropriate to their status. An ambassadorial report written in 1565, during the pontificate of Pius IV, when the spirit of the Council of Trent found full embodiment in the papacy, is revealing of these considerations. The report informs us regarding the climate at the papal court at the time: simplicity, morality and maintaining a distance from amusements constituted the ideal that cardinals and their courtiers ought to follow, at least in public.[29]

In the endeavour of the Catholic Church to support moral and spiritual reform, particular dances were singled out for denunciation due to moral, religious and theological considerations.[30] The *moresca* was criticized by the religious authorities as vulgar, disorderly and deviant. It was said to threaten the social order, while the papal Church aspired from its representatives (and their courtiers) strict norms of behaviour and conduct as well as complete order in everyday lifestyle, so as to set the example for the rest of the flock. Nonetheless, while advocates of the Catholic Reformation attacked excess and lack of decorum, overall, their goal was not the abolition of occasions for dance; rather, they aimed for its modification and purification according to the new standards.[31] It was not the body activity per se that was criticized; rather, it was the purpose and the circumstances under which a body activity was practiced that defined it as appropriate or not. In this framework, the *locus* of the body discourse was shifting from the body to the soul and the emphasis was set on the intention of body practices.

27 For Cardinal Alessandro Farnese as Rome's most important individual patron, see Robertson, *'Il Gran Cardinale'*.

28 Burke, *Popular Culture*, p. 213.

29 Robertson, *'Il Gran Cardinale'*, pp. 75-76.

30 Burke, *Popular Culture*, pp. 209-212.

31 Ibid., p. 215.

Moderating the extraordinary moresca through medicine and the ancient example

The Counter-Reformation sought the Christianization of body culture through the implementation of the principles of moderation, restraint, order and control. These principles served as the guiding lines in the practice of a series of body activities, daily and festive, and shaped the attitudes towards body culture overall, especially on the part of the representatives of the papal Church. In the framework of the Counter-Reformation, this moral-religious discourse significantly influenced other discourses and often overlapped with the medical discourse; furthermore, it involved the whole community rather than the individual alone, and along with medicine, it played a major role in contemporary policies of social control.

Mercuriale's *De arte gymnastica* responds to these moral-religious aspirations and the shifting attitudes towards the exceptional body. Indicatively, in Book III, Chapter I, 'De agendis et de ratione praesentis tractationis' (Our agenda and the rationale behind this treatise), drawing from Plato's *Timaeus*, Mercuriale asserts that

> gymnastics, although it may appear to concern itself solely with the body, also treats body and soul together, as Plato recommended in his *Timaeus*, so that it does not allow the body to rampage insolently in its toughness and strength, but subjects it to the domination, control and direction of the rational activities of the soul [anima].[32]

Similarly, in Book I, Chapter IV, 'De gymnastica subiecto er eius laudibus' (The subject of gymnastics and its reputation), Mercuriale, drawing from Plato's *Protagoras*, claims that 'the person who only exercises his soul, while sloth and inactivity consume his body, deserves to be called a cripple'.[33]

Mercuriale's medical discourse on dance and the *moresca* is an enlightening historical example of how body culture was modified through medicine in order to fit contemporary political-religious criteria of appropriate, regulated and moderate body movement. After all, dance was classified as a physical exercise and its health benefits were the subject matter of medical treatises, especially of preventive medicine and the literature of general well-being. Physicians explored the role of dance in maintaining

32 DAG, p. 323.
33 Ibid., p. 35.

health as well as its being a cause, symptom or remedy for disease.[34] Although its beneficial role as a physical exercise was rarely challenged, the strong moral notions regarding dance prevailed in the medical discourse as well; physicians indicated excessive and disordered dance both to be a cause of disease as well as a disease itself. In a similar manner, Mercuriale examines dance from a medical point of view. He notes that the principles that should pertain to dance – and body activity in general – in order to be considered a medical exercise, and therefore have a medical effect and value, are moderation, order, control and measure. In addition, dance should be practiced only for medical reasons and according to the physician's advice regarding the right occasion and time in the day and the right place (e.g. the Greco-Roman *palaestra* or gymnasium, which was an open space dedicated for training, exercise and sport). Otherwise, it could be the cause of disease.[35]

Mercuriale dedicates four chapters of his *De arte gymnastica* to dance.[36] In Book II, Chapter III, 'De saltatoria' (The saltatory), Mercuriale identifies the *saltatory* ('dance' in Latin) as one of the two parts of medical gymnastics and he asserts its medical value in the maintenance and obtainment of health. Following the medical authority of Galen, Mercuriale claims that dance was a part of medical gymnastics and that Galen 'restored good health to many feeble patients by means of wrestling, the pankratium, dance and similar exercises'.[37] Mercuriale notes that

> no one should doubt that we have properly included dance in the category of gymnastic medicine, especially since Socrates in the *Symposium* of Xenophon openly declares that he had practiced dancing with a view to both achieving and maintaining health and also to acquire strength of body.[38]

He also notes that 'Galen regarded dancers' training as one of the things sought after by doctors'.[39]

In Book V, Chapter III, 'De saltatoriae effectibus' (The effects of the saltatory), examining the medical effects and value of dance, Mercuriale

34 Alessandro Arcangeli has written extensively for the role of dance in early modern medicine, as a physical exercise. See Arcangeli, 'Dance and Health'; Arcangeli, *Recreation*.

35 DAG, bk IV, chaps X, XI, XII, XIII.

36 DAG, bk II, chap. III, 'The Saltatory'; chap. VI, 'Dancing or the Third Part of the Saltatory'; chap. VII, 'The Purpose and Place of Dancing'; bk V, chap. III, 'The Effects of the Saltatory'.

37 DAG, p. 223. The *pankration* was an ancient athletic sporting event that involved both boxing and wrestling.

38 Ibid.

39 Ibid., p. 255.

compares ancient dance culture to contemporary dance culture. He notes that when one looks at the various types of the ancient forebears' dances, they will see that 'they were not lacking in rhythm, pattern, proportion and musical harmony'.[40] Musical harmony was an expression of the *misura* (measure, 'moderation' in Latin) that indicated proportion and order that were sought in the connection of movement with sound.[41] The role of music was crucial: measure, rhythm, the beat of the music, and the timing of the steps, were accepted by all (dance masters, writers, etc.) as fundamental to dancing.[42]

Mercuriale criticizes the dance culture of his contemporaries. He observes that

> [c]onsequently it can be supposed that our own dances, cavortings, and gestures, which are enjoyed nowadays both by women and by men, in pursuit of delight and pleasure, differed from the dances of the ancients in this way: the latter often were good for the preservation of health, whereas ours seldom or never have that end in view. On the contrary, they are indulged in, mostly, after dinner and by night, as part of the banquet – at an hour when sleep and rest would be much better.[43]

Mercuriale claims that '[s]o it is that dancing, if only it were practiced at the right time, as it was by our ancestors, and as we have already shown that all exercises ought to be, would undeniably be productive of many advantages.[44] Furthermore, in Book II, Chapter VII, 'De fine saltationis et de loco' (The purpose and place of dancing), Mercuriale notes that

> indeed, in our own times no one would deny that other dances performed in time, formation, and a prescribed way, would have such utility, inductive to good deportment and the maintenance of health, just as Galen declares that he had restored many to health, and he had maintained others in health by the art of dance alone.[45]

Through this comparison between ancient and contemporary dance culture, Mercuriale defines the preconditions that are necessary for dance to be

40 Ibid., p. 543.
41 Nevile, *The Eloquent Body*, pp. 77-82.
42 McGowan, *Dance*, pp. 39-40.
43 DAG, p. 545.
44 Ibid.
45 Ibid., p. 255.

considered a medical exercise. He distinguishes ancient from contemporary dance practices in terms of intention and purpose as well as in terms of the circumstances under which dance should be practiced. According to Mercuriale, contemporary dance habits, contrary to the ancient ones, aim for the pursuit of delight and pleasure rather than health; they involve indulgence, they lack in rhythm, proportion, and harmony, and they are practiced at the wrong time (i.e. after eating, in a banquet, late at night). In these terms, contemporary dance culture, according to Mercuriale, implies disorder, lack of control, moderation and decorum; thus, it is harmful for health and deviant in terms of conduct. On the other side of the argument, ancient dancing can be considered beneficial for health, if it is practiced for medical reasons only, in the right time, with moderation, measure, control, order, as well as formation and rhythm (and with musical harmony).

Here, the medical discourse overlaps with the moral-religious discourse. On the one hand, notions of the healthy body overlap with notions of the ordered, controlled, moderated body. On the other hand, the unhealthy body overlaps with the deviant body, which lacks order, control and moderation. It is crucial to consider that in the period under examination there was an emphasis on the measured and controlled movement of one's body that was shared by the religious authorities, humanists and dance masters, indicating a widespread concern regarding the control of one's body.[46] Such a movement was considered the outward sign of a person's moral nature. It implied that the person who could control their outward body movements could control their inner emotions as well. Moderation, order and temperance in everyday life activities were a prerequisite for the post-Tridentine (i.e. after the Council of Trent) Catholic Church; activities had to be controlled and conformed to a set of rules and standards. Moderation in movement, in particular, was highly valued by humanists, dance masters and physicians alike; in this they drew from Aristotle's teachings and the Latin rhetorical texts that stressed the importance of moderation in relation to virtue and eloquent movement. Eloquent movement was considered an outward manifestation of the movements of a person's soul, whereas vulgar movements were a sign that a person's soul was not virtuous and was out of harmony with the world.[47] Mercuriale's medical discourse reflects these considerations as he suggests that ordered and controlled, moderate body movement in dance is an essential prerequisite for a healthy body and a moral soul.

46 Nevile, *The Eloquent Body*, p. 90.
47 Ibid., p. 91.

The fact that in his *De arte gymnastica* Mercuriale explores body practices of ancient origin has an essential significance and is revealing for the purposes of the present essay. The ancient body culture – and antiquity in general – was a major humanist interest and fascination of sixteenth-century Roman court culture. Cardinal Alessandro Farnese himself owned an impressive private collection of antiquities. However, in the era after the Council of Trent, the Catholic reformers put antiquity under scrutiny and criticized it as too worldly, pagan and unchristian. In his medical discourse, Mercuriale manages to moderate the controversial ancient body culture by attributing to it a medical and a broader moral value. In *De arte gymnastica* ancient dance culture is promoted as an *exemplum* ('example' in Latin).[48] Mercuriale emphasizes the positive characteristics of ancient dance culture and he makes a moral argument, promoting it as an example, a model to be followed, by demonstrating that it followed the principles of order, measure, control and decorum. Here again, the moral-religious discourse and the medical discourse overlap: the religious-moral principles advocated by the Catholic Reformation are indicated by Mercuriale (and the medical teaching at the time) as the necessary preconditions for dance – and for other body activities – to have a medical value and effect. By bringing forward ancient dancing as exemplary, Mercuriale connected dance to health, temperance, harmony and virtue.

In the same framework of comparison between antiquity and his own time, in Book II, Chapter III, 'De saltatoria' (The saltatory), Mercuriale, following the medical authority of Galen, examines the dance known as *intermedio*, which from the late fifteenth century onwards was identified with *moresca*.[49] He notes that 'the dance known as *intermedio*, which by nature stands between round dance and shadow-fighting, can be performed by children, women and old men who have feeble as well as thin bodies'. Drawing from Plato, he writes, 'I dare say that we may be dealing with that class of dance which Plato calls irenic or appropriate to peaceful times and which he writes is performed in times of prosperity giving moderate pleasure to temperate souls.'[50] Here again, Mercuriale highlights the principles of moderation and temperance.

In Book II, Chapter VI, 'De orchestica sive tertia saltatoriae parte' (Dancing or the third part of the saltatory), Mercuriale identifies the

48 Alessandro Arcangeli has written on *exempla* (plural for *exemplum*), which were narratives used as rhetorical devices and means of persuasion of moral instruction on dance. See Arcangeli, 'Dance and Punishment'. On the tradition of *exempla* associated with ancient and medieval literary genres, see Maja Bondestam's chapter on prodigious bodies ('An Education') in this volume.

49 Nevile, *The Eloquent Body*, pp. 34-34.

50 DAG, p. 223.

origins of the *moresca* in the ancient Greek martial dance known as the 'Pyrrhic'. He points the reader's attention to an illustration of the Pyrrhic featured in his book,[51] writing 'armed men dance sometimes chanting and sometimes in silence, as can be seen from this image from some ancient stones, which we have printed here'. In the following, he notes that 'in our day the equivalent of the Pyrrhic dances are the sort of mock combats that are popularly known as *morescas*'.[52] Mercuriale's fascination with the Pyrrhic was common in his time and was indicative of the broader humanist fascination with antiquity. Furthermore, the interest in the Pyrrhic emerges as highly relevant to Mercuriale's contemporary dance types, as its form had distinct affinities with both imitative and geometrical patterns of dancing.

Mercuriale, drawing from Plutarch's 'Table Talk IX', locates the practice of the Pyrrhic in the space of the *palaestra* and he points out its valorous style and its value in military training. He notes that

> to the point that our ancestors practiced the art of dance to acquire bodily strength and equally military skill, for which it is approved by Plato, must be added the further point that an armed dance, called Pyrrhic, was invented for no other purpose than to allow, through its valorous style, boys as well as women to learn how at one time to evade the enemy at another to attack and also other activities necessary in the conduct of war.[53]

In addition, Mercuriale emphasizes the pedagogical and medical value of the Pyrrhic. He notes that

> it is easy to assert that this same dance was immensely conducive to good deportment and the maintenance of health, since the subject of hand gestures or hand control is discussed both by Hippocrates and by Aretaeus, and is deployed by others with regard to the exercise of bodies in health and sometimes in illness too.[54]

51 The illustration of the Pyrrhic and the majority of the illustrations featured in the *De arte gymnastica* were added in the second edition of the book (Venice, 1573). The drawings were courtesy of the artist, architect and antiquarian Pirro Ligorio (1513-1583). Girolamo Mercuriale and Pirro Ligorio moved in the same circles while they were both residents in Rome, with Ligorio living there for more than 25 years before Mercuriale arrived in 1562. For the illustrations in the *De arte gymnastica*, see DAG, pp. 863-872.

52 DAG., p. 251.

53 Ibid., p. 255.

54 Ibid.

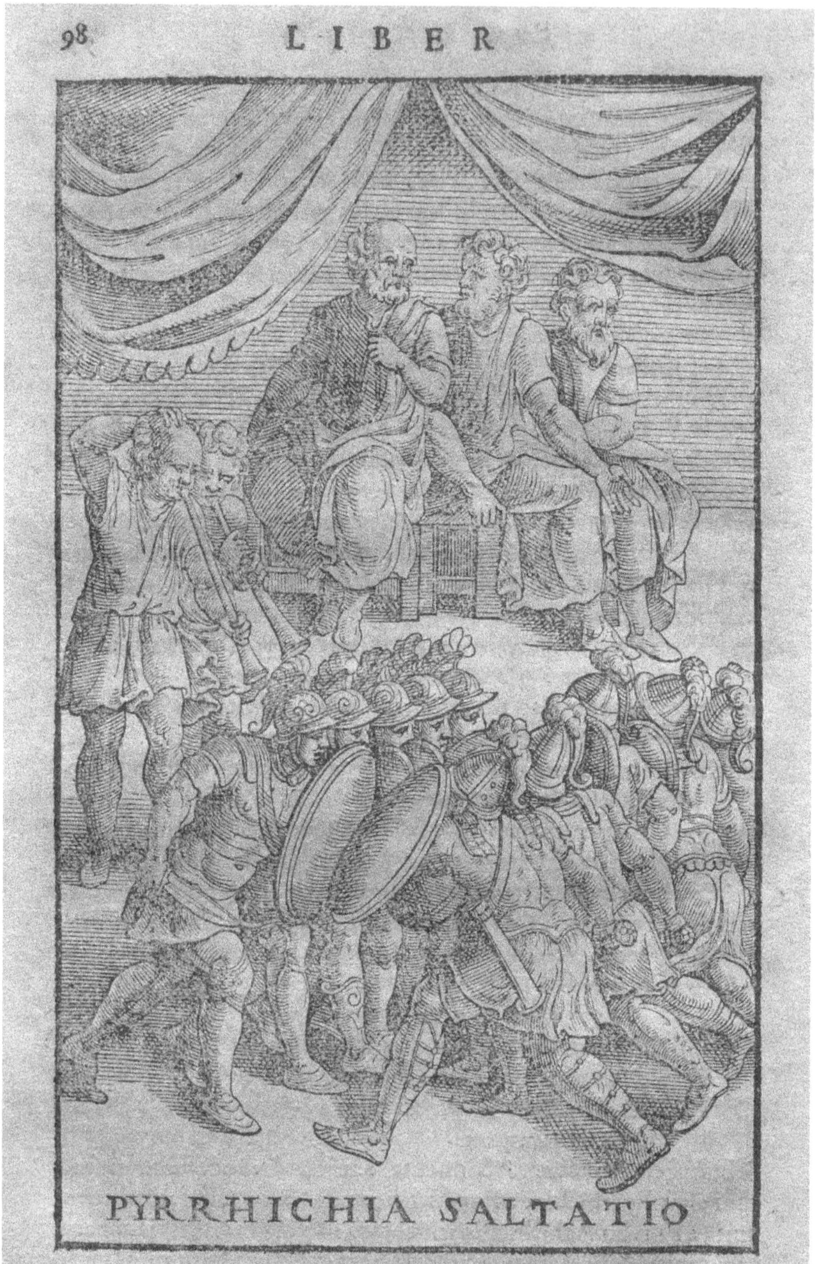

Figure 1.1. Pirro Ligorio, *Pyrrhichia saltatio* [The Pyrrhic dance], 1573. Engraving from Girolamo Mercuriale, *De arte gymnastica Libri sex, in quibus exercitationum omnium vetustarum genera, loca, modi, facultates & quidquid deniq. Ad corporis humani exeritationes pertinent, diligenter explicatur. Secunda editione, aucti, et multis figuris ornati* (Venetiis [Venezia], Apud Iuntas, 1573), VI, p. 98. Biblioteca Nazionale Centrale di Roma, Rome. Photograph: Uppsala University Library.

In fact, what was stressed in Mercuriale's time was the ancient origin of this dance as well as the skill and agility required to perform a dance with such complex gestures and movements.[55]

We see therefore that in Mercuriale's discourse the *moresca*, which made part of the elite's rituals of public display and private celebrations manifesting the fascination in the extraordinary and the wondrous bodies, is moderated in two ways. First, the *moresca* is identified with the ancient *exemplum*, that is, the Pyrrhic. In this way, it acquires ancient origin, indigenous nature, as well as moral and pedagogical value as, according to Mercuriale, the Pyrrhic contributes to good comportment, body temperance, order and control. Second, it is modified into a medical exercise as, according to Mercuriale, it can be used for the maintenance of health and the treatment of disease when practiced in the proper way, time and place. Here again, the medical and the moral-religious discourse overlap as far as the notions of morality and health are concerned. As the spectacle of the extraordinary and wondrous bodies is modified into a medical exercise with ancient origin in Mercuriale's medical discourse, the shift in the nature, purpose, place and time of the *moresca* becomes evident: its nature shifts from a 'danced drama' to a medical exercise; its purpose shifts from causing wonder, awe and amusement to exercising the body, offering moderate pleasure, building strength and assisting in military training; the exaggerated movements and gestures of the dancers shift to ordered, controlled and measured movement of the exercising body; from public and private spectacles of display, festivities, etc. its practice moves to controlled spaces for exercising (i.e. the *palaestra*).

The illustration of the Pyrrhic featured in the book further serves Mercuriale's endeavour to moderate the extraordinary *moresca* through the ancient example. The illustrations featured in early modern scientific and medical books served practical purposes as they conveyed instantly what the text takes more time to describe, as well as aesthetic and decorative purposes. Nonetheless, illustrations – just like text – raise problems of context, function, rhetoric, recollection (whether soon or long after the event featured), second-hand witnessing and so on.[56] In the case of Mercuriale's *De arte gymnastica*, the antiquarian origin and styling of the illustration undoubtedly serve to document the ancient remains and objects that Mercuriale used as his sources. In this way, the illustration functions as a form of historical evidence and, as such, a means of persuading his audience that

55 McGowan, *Dance*, pp. 124-126.

56 Burke, *Eyewitnessing*, p. 15.

what he is writing and arguing about is 'true', since at the time the ancient classical sources (primarily the textual and secondarily the material) were the absolute authority of true knowledge.

Nonetheless, at the same time the illustration portraying the Pyrrhic represents and visualizes the ancient example that Mercuriale promotes: the dance type that was pertained by the principles of order, control and measure, and as such led to a body and soul that are orderly, controlled and, thus, healthy. The illustration visualizes for the readers of the *De arte gymnastica* the shift in the features of the *moresca* that Mercuriale attempts as he identifies it with the ancient Pyrrhic: the element of the grotesque, the special effects, the exotic characters, the monstrous bodies, the blackened figures, the savages, the barbarians, the wild men, the strange and the outlandish elements that constituted the exceptional and the extraordinary nature of the *moresca* are eliminated in this picture. What is visualized in Mercuriale's endeavour to moderate the *moresca*, is the ancient robust, athletic male bodies wearing armour and engaging in mock combat, in perfect alignment and order and in a rather unadorned setting.

We see therefore that Mercuriale's endeavour to moderate, to regulate exceptional and wondrous bodies that were an essential part of a well-established court lifestyle and etiquette, goes through medicine and antiquarianism. It is articulated around a series of medical and moral-religious principles, the notion of the familiar and the indigenous (i.e. the Greco-Roman origin) as opposed to the 'exotic', and the authoritative Greco-Roman past as visualized in the illustration of the Pyrrhic featured in the *De arte gymnastica*, which is promoted as exemplary in both medical and moral terms. In Mercuriale's medical discourse, the *moresca* is modified from a custom and spectacle of extraordinary corporeality into a regulated, moderate body practice with medical benefits, based on the values of temperance, control and order in accordance with the religious-moral criteria of the Catholic Church.

Conclusion

The present essay suggests that Mercuriale's *De arte gymnastica* is an important historical source that reveals tensions and shifting attitudes towards body culture, as they were manifested in the context of court medicine in Counter-Reformation Rome. Mercuriale's medical discourse on dance and the *moresca* throws light on the medical, moral and religious tensions that courtly fascination with extraordinary bodies and body practices raised. It shows how the Roman (mostly ecclesiastical) elite's fascination with exceptional bodies and spectacles of wonder had to be consolidated with the aspirations for spiritual reform raised by the Counter-Reformation papacy, that went hand in hand with bodily reform. This was in a time when the Catholic Church condemned dance as disordered due to connections to a vulgar, disharmonic, mischievous and unhealthy body and soul and targeted the behaviour of its clergy trying to direct its flock towards spiritual reform as a way to deal with the protestant 'heresy'. In this charged environment, Mercuriale moderates the controversial *moresca* through medicine and the ancient example, demonstrating its virtuous aspects when practiced for medical reasons, in the right time, with temperance, measure, control, formation, rhythm and order. In this way, the extraordinary *moresca* is regulated in accordance with the aspirations of the Catholic reformers.

In Mercuriale's medical discourse the values of temperance, control and order (shared by both medical and religious authorities) that should pertain to body movement, conduct and lifestyle in general, emerge as the crucial principles for moderating the extraordinary and deviant body. Particularly in dance, order was considered to lead towards moral virtue. Order and geometric shapes in choreography represented the order of the cosmos, while geometrical movement in dance was thought to encourage men and women to imitate the divine order in their lives through noble and virtuous behaviour.[57] Temperance in movement signified a virtuous soul, a person who is not dominated either by excess of vice or by excessive virtue. On the contrary, excessive movement (or no movement at all) was a sign of a disordered body and a soul full of moral flaws.[58] After all, according to the definition of dance that Mercuriale provides in Book II, Chapter VI, 'De orchestica sive tertia saltatoriae parte' (Dancing or the third part of the saltatory), dance is 'the faculty of imitating character, affections and actions by deliberately artful and rhythmical movements and gestures'.[59] He notes that pointing with the arms and imitation in dancing suggest the 'rhythmical and ordered movements of the earth, sky or the surroundings'.[60] In this way, dance reflected a bond between body and soul, but also between macrocosmic and microcosmic orders in the Counter-Reformation era.

57 Nevile, *The Eloquent Body*, p. 11.
58 Ibid., p. 10.
59 DAG, p. 247.
60 Ibid., p. 249.

Furthermore, Mercuriale's medical discourse on dance and the *moresca* reveals the shifting attitudes of the early modern elites towards exceptional and wondrous bodies. As Daston and Park note, the wonder migrated during the early modern period 'from the pole of awed reverence to that of dull, stupor, becoming the ruling passion of the vulgar mob rather than of the philosophical elite'.[61] The elite separated themselves from the vulgar in their ability to distinguish things that were truly 'wonderful' from things that were not. They also set cultural boundaries between the domestic and the exotic and between the cultivated and the vulgar.[62]

In this regard, we should highlight three points. First, Mercuriale's attempt to locate and identify the origins of the *moresca* in the exemplary, domestic, ancient Greco-Roman past. Second, Mercuriale's antiquarianism. In the *De arte gymnastica* antiquarianism, a growing field and method of learning that was flourishing in Rome and was congenial to medicine as well,[63] enriches the study of the nature of the *moresca* as a noble body practice and upgrades it to a subject matter of intellectual inquiry for his learned elite audience. Third, Mercuriale's remarks that in his own day 'dancing had become perverted [...] and had descended from its lofty position to hold tyrannical sway over tumultuous and ignorant audiences; every good man knows that this habit has persisted even to our own day when all dancing has become corrupted'.[64] Popular at both courts and markets, the *moresca* reveals tensions between the learned social elite on the one hand and the unlearned laity on the other, who were supposed to have corrupted it. The possibility of the abuse of dance by the ignorant (i.e. the unlearned) was a common argument that clerics and moralists employed in the Counter-Reformation era. It was considered that when dance was abused by the unlearned, it might have negative effects, whereas when practiced by virtuous and noble men who were informed about its style, structure and philosophical framework, it only had positive results and beneficial effects.[65]

Mercuriale's *De arte gymnastica* could be read as the endeavour of a humanist court physician to moderate exceptional, extraordinary bodies in a time when the social, political and religious circumstances required

61 Daston and Park, *Wonders*, p. 305.

62 Ibid., p. 20.

63 For the flourishing of antiquarianism in Rome and its affiliations with humanist medicine, see Siraisi, *History, Medicine*.

64 DAG, p. 249.

65 Nevile, *The Eloquent Body*, p. 68.

modification and regulation of body culture as a whole. By transforming the *moresca* into a (bodily and moral) health-bringing exercise with ancient connotations and a learned background, Mercuriale suggests that the *moresca* was not vulgar. Daston and Park argue that similar changes in the field of extraordinary wonders was 'a profound mutation in the self-definition of intellectuals'.[66] Wonders faded from prominence in elite circles but still were, according to Daston and Park, in the late seventeenth century partly constitutive of what it meant to be part of a cultural elite in Europe.[67] The complexities in the history of exceptional bodies and wonders seen in the context of early modern court dance culture, which embodied nuanced social-political value and connotations, should, it seems, be taken seriously. The *De arte gymnastica* demonstrates the physician's endeavour to bring exceptional bodies and social-cultural practices that were well-rooted in the early modern world, under control according to the demands of the political-religious authorities. It becomes evident that learned medicine – even in the early modern period – had a much wider remit than merely providing cures.[68]

Works Cited

Primary Sources

Mercuriale, Girolamo, *Arte ginnastica*, trans. Ippolito Galante (Rome: Banco di Santo Spirito, 1960).

Mercuriale, Girolamo, *Artis gymnasticae apud antiquos celeberrimae, nostris ignoratae, libri sex In quibus exercitationum omnium vetustarum genera, loca, modi, facultates et quicquid denique ad corporis humani exercitationes pertinet, diligenter explicatur. Opus non modo medicis, verum etiam omnibus antiquarum rerum cognoscendarum et valetudinis conservandae studiosis admondum utile. Auctore Hieronymo Mercuriali Foroliviensi Medico et Philosopho. Medico & Philosopho* (Venetiis [Venezia], Apud Iuntas, In officina Iuntarum, MDLXIX [1569]).

Mercuriale, Girolamo, *De arte gymnastica*, ed. and trans. Michele Napolitano; introduction by Robert Stalla (Rome: Edizioni Elefante, 1996).

Mercuriale, Girolamo, *De arte gymnastica*, ed. Concetta Pennuto, trans. Vivian Nutton (Firenze: Leo S. Olschki, 2008).

66 Daston and Park, *Wonders*, p. 18.

67 Ibid., p. 19.

68 Wear, *Knowledge and Practice*, p. 155.

Mercuriale, Girolamo, *De arte gymnastica Libri sex, in quibus exercitationum omnium vetustarum genera, loca, modi, facultates & quidquid deniq. Ad corporis humani exeritationes pertinent, diligenter explicatur. Secunda editione, aucti, et multis figuris ornati* (Venetiis [Venezia], Apud Iuntas, MDLXXIII [1573]), seconda edizione dopo quella di Venezia del 1569.

Mercuriale, Girolamo, *L'Art de la gymnastique. Livre premier/De arte gymnastica. Liber primus*, ed., trans., presentation and notes by Jean-Michel Agasse (Paris: Les Belles Lettres, 2006).

Secondary Sources

Arcangeli, Alessandro, 'Dance and Health: The Renaissance Physician's View', *Dance Research: The Journal of the Society for Dance Research* 18, no. 1 (2000), pp. 3-30.

Arcangeli, Alessandro, 'Dance and Punishment', *Dance Research: The Journal of the Society for Dance Research* 10, no. 2 (1992), pp. 30-42.

Arcangeli, Alessandro, 'Dance under Trial: The Moral Debate 1200-1600', *Dance Research: The Journal of the Society for Dance Research* 12, no. 2 (1994), pp. 127-155.

Arcangeli, Alessandro, 'Dancing Savages: Stereotypes and Cultural Encounters across the Atlantic in the Age of European Expansion', in *Exploring Cultural History: Essays in Honour of Peter Burke*, ed. Melissa Calaresu, Filippo De Vivo and Joan-Pau Rubiés (Farnham: Ashgate, 2010), pp. 289-308.

Arcangeli, Alessandro, *Recreation in the Renaissance: Attitudes towards Leisure and Pastimes in European Culture, c. 1425-1675* (Hampshire: Palgrave Macmillan, 2003).

Bourdieu, Pierre, *Language and Symbolic Power* (Cambridge: Polity Press, 1994).

Burke, Peter, *Eyewitnessing: The Uses of Images as Historical Evidence* (London: Reaktion Books, 2001).

Burke, Peter, *Popular Culture in Early Modern Europe* (London: Harper Torchbooks, 1978).

Cavallo, Sandra, and Tessa Storey, *Healthy Living in Late Renaissance Italy* (Oxford: Oxford University Press, 2013).

Daston, Lorraine, and Katharine Park, *Wonders and the Order of Nature, 1150-1750* (New York: Zone Books, 1998).

Forrest, John, *History of Morris Dancing, 1458-1750* (Toronto: University of Toronto Press, 1999).

Foucault, Michel, *Archaeology of Knowledge and the Discourse on Language*, trans. A.M. Sheridan Smith (New York: Pantheon Books, 1972).

Geertz, Clifford, 'Thick Description: Toward an Interpretative Theory of Culture', in *The Interpretation of Cultures: Selected Essays*, ed. Clifford Geertz (New York: Basic Books, 1973), pp. 3-32

Godden, Richard H., 'Embodied Difference: Monstrosity, Disability, and the Posthuman', in *Monstrosity, Disability, and the Posthuman in the Medieval and Early Modern World,* ed. Richard H. Godden and Asa Simon Mittman (Cham: Palgrave Macmillan, 2019), pp. 3-31.

Locke, Ralph P., *Music and the Exotic from the Renaissance to Mozart* (Cambridge: Cambridge University Press, 2015).

McClelland, John, and Brian Merrilees, *Sport and Culture in Early Modern Europe*, ed. John McClelland and Brian Merrilees (Toronto: Centre for Reformation and Renaissance Studies, 2009).

McGinnis, Katherine, *Moving in High Circles: Courts, Dances and Dancing Masters in Italy in the Long Sixteenth Century* (Ann Arbor: University Microfilms International, 2001).

McGowan, Margaret M., *Dance in the Renaissance: European Fashion, French Obsession* (New Haven: Yale University Press, 2008).

Nevile, Jennifer, *The Eloquent Body: Dance and Humanist Culture in Fifteenth-Century Italy* (Bloomington: Indiana University Press, 2004).

Pušnik, Maruša, 'Introduction: Dance as Social Life and Cultural Practice', *Anthropological Notebooks* 16, no. 3 (2010), pp. 5-8.

Radcliffe-Brown, A.R., and E.E. Evans-Pritchard, *Structure and Function in Primitive Society: Essays and Addresses* (New York: The Free Press, 1952).

Rizzi, Alessandra, 'Regulated Play at the End of the Middle Ages: The Work of Mendicant Preachers in Communal Italy', in *Sport and Culture in Early Modern Europe*, ed. John McClelland and Brian Merrilees (Toronto: Centre for Reformation and Renaissance Studies, 2009), pp. 41-69.

Robertson, Clare, *'Il Gran Cardinale': Alessandro Farnese, Patron of the Arts* (New Haven: Yale University Press, 1992).

Siraisi, Nancy G., *History, Medicine, and the Traditions of Renaissance Learning* (Ann Arbor: University of Michigan Press, 2007).

Sparti, Barbara, 'The Function and Status of Dance in the Fifteenth-Century Italian Courts', *Dance Research: The Journal of the Society for Dance Research* 14, no. 1 (1996), pp. 42-61.

Sparti, Barbara, 'Part I, Introduction, Chapter 3 'Dancing in Fifteenth-Cntury Italian Society', in Guglielmo Ebreo of Pesaro, *De Pratica seu Arte Tripudii/On the Practice or Art of Dancing*, ed. and trans. Barbara Sparti. Poems trans. Michael Sullivan (Oxford: Oxford University Press, 1993), pp. 47-62.

Sutton, Richard L., Jr, *Sixteenth Century Physician and His Methods: Mercurialis on Diseases of the Skin* (Kansas City: The Lowell Press, 1986).

Wear, Andrew, *Knowledge and Practice in English Medicine, 1550-1680* (Cambridge: Cambridge University Press, 2000).

About the Author

Maria Kavvadia holds a PhD diploma from the Department of History and Civilization of the European University Institute. Her research interests mainly lie in the area of early modern scientific cultures and knowledge traditions, cultural practices in science and medicine, court medicine, body culture, and scientific and medical illustration.

2. Monsters and the Maternal Imagination: The 'First Vision' from Johann Remmelin's 1619 *Catoptrum microcosmicum* Triptych

Rosemary Moore

Abstract
The 'First Vision' of Johann Remmelin's 1619 print triptych, *Catoptrum microcosmicum* (Mirrors of the microcosm) teems with allegorical and biblical emblems, alongside anatomical illustrations. This chapter focuses on the serpent-haired creature that obscures the genitals of a pregnant torso. The juxtaposition implies an affinity between the monstrous and the maternal that is paralleled in early modern conceptions of the maternal imagination. However, that affinity is far from straightforward. The print belongs to an innovative category of anatomical illustration known as the 'fugitive sheet'. As such it employs carefully cut and pasted layers to reproduce the spatiality of the body or organ depicted. Moving through those layers, a number of surprising features are revealed, unsettling the apparent symmetry and stability of the design.

Keywords: anatomical fugitive sheet, anatomy, Medusa, *Mirrors of the Microcosm*, pregnancy

An extraordinary flame-eared creature with hair like that of Medusa – a tangled nest of serpents – obstructs visual access to the secrets of the pregnant body in the 'First Vision' of Johann Remmelin's *Catoptrum microcosmicum* (Mirrors of the microcosm) triptych (Augsburg: Davidis Francki, 1619) (fig. 2.1). The strategic overlaying of this monstrous creature against the heavily distended form of a truncated, female torso implies an affinity between the monstrous and the maternal. But the nature of this

Bondestam, M. (ed.), *Exceptional Bodies in Early Modern Culture: Concepts of Monstrosity before the Advent of the Normal*. Taylor & Francis Group, 2020
DOI 10.5117/9789463721745_CH02

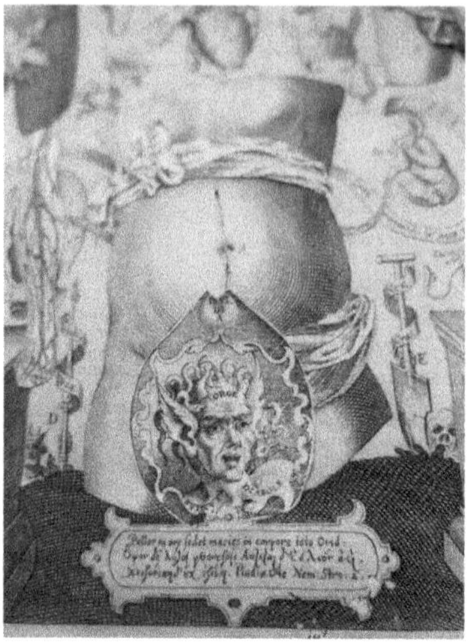

Figure 2.1. Detail of the monstrous creature in Johann Remmelin, 'First Vision', 1619. Etching and engraving from *Catoptrum microcosmicum*. Wellcome Library, London. Photograph: Rosemary Moore.

affinity remains ambiguous. Is the creature intended to mark the female body as something ugly, dangerous or corrupting even? Does it represent the unruly powers of the maternal imagination? Or could it function as an apotropaic shield, guarding against the licentious gazes of both the beholder and the beheld? Moreover, what – if any – is the significance of the peculiar resemblance between this creature and the mythical gorgon, Medusa?

Monsters were, of course, closely associated with the maternal body and the imagination in early modern culture. Scholars such as Marie Hélène Huet, Lorraine Daston and Katharine Park have shown that monstrous births were widely believed to be the direct consequence of a pregnant woman's highly susceptible, and therefore dangerous, imagination.[1] Yet this issue has received little attention in relation to Remmelin's 'First Vision'.[2] Instead, scholarly interest has focused on the apparent oppositions that, it is argued, bring stability and order to an otherwise baffling array of emblems, all of which vie for attention on the printed page. For although today the *Catoptrum microcosmicum* triptych is usually defined as anatomical illustration, its surfaces teem with allegorical and religious messages alongside representations of the human

1 Daston and Park, *Wonders*; Huet, *Monstrous Imagination*.

2 Lyle Massey comments briefly on the potential for the creature to function as an apotropaic device related to pregnancy. See Massey, 'The Alchemical Womb', p. 221.

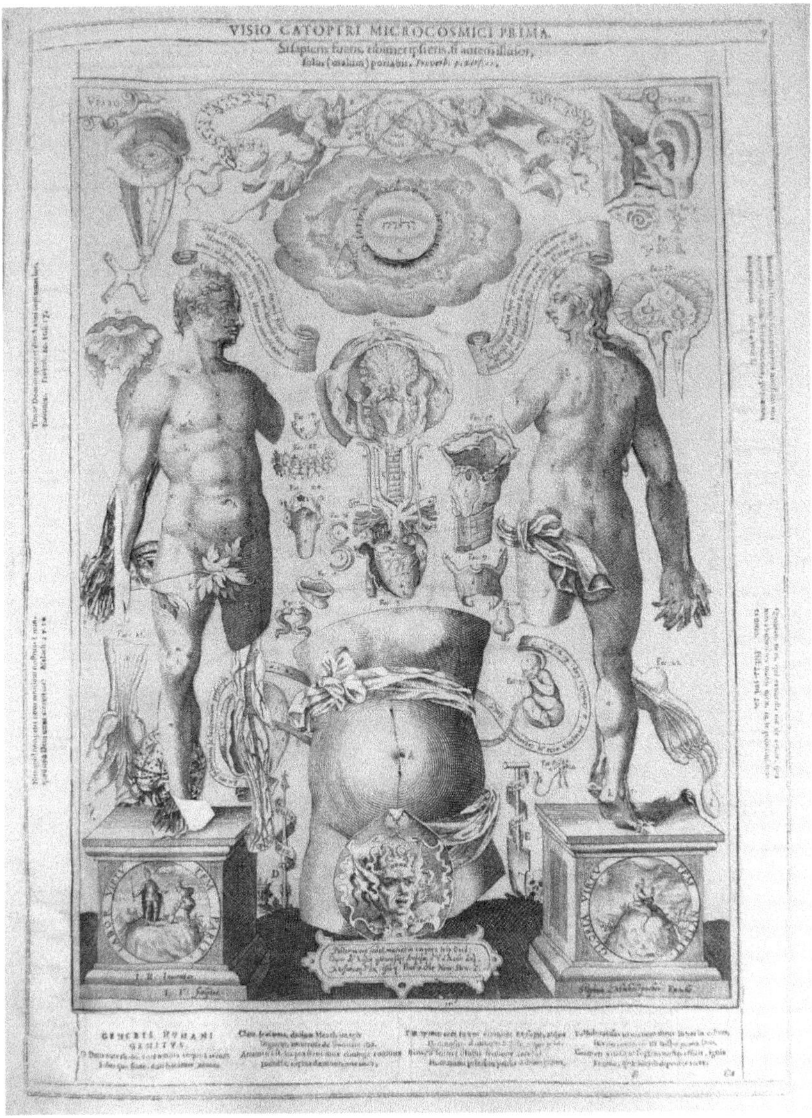

Figure 2.2. Johann Remmelin, 'First Vision', 1619. Etching and engraving from *Catoptrum microcosmicum*. Wellcome Library, London. Photograph: Rosemary Moore.

body's internal organs (figs 2.2, 2.3, 2.4). The nineteenth-century physician and medical historian Ludwig Choulant was particularly scathing in his analysis of this, stating that: 'The anatomic value of these drawings is very slight and even as a whole, they represent the clumsiest study of anatomy.'[3]

3 Choulant, *History*, p. 232.

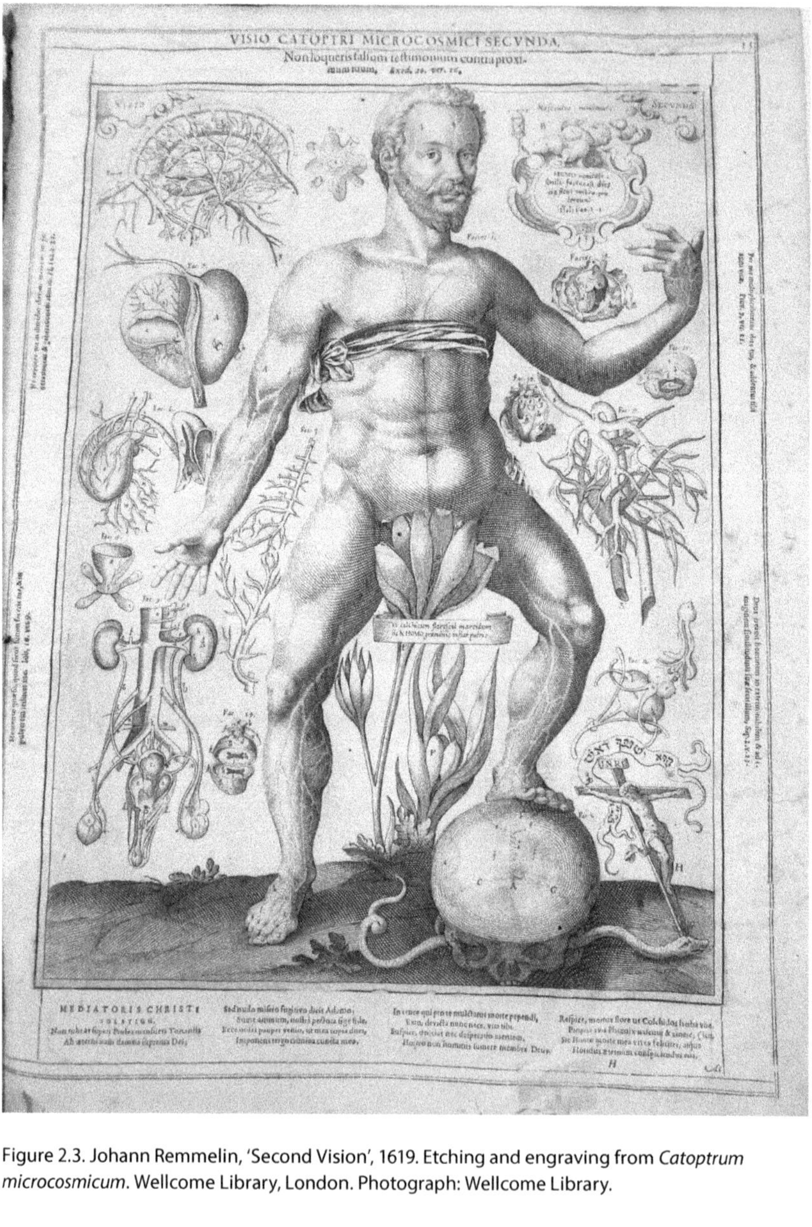

Figure 2.3. Johann Remmelin, 'Second Vision', 1619. Etching and engraving from *Catoptrum microcosmicum*. Wellcome Library, London. Photograph: Wellcome Library.

Recent scholarly attention has been somewhat more generous. For David Hillman and Carla Mazzio, the prints are not 'clumsy' but actually employ sophisticated strategies aimed at holding bodily knowledge together.[4] The dominant strategy they identify is one of oppositions: male/female, inside/

4 Hillman and Mazzio, 'Introduction', pp. xv-xvi.

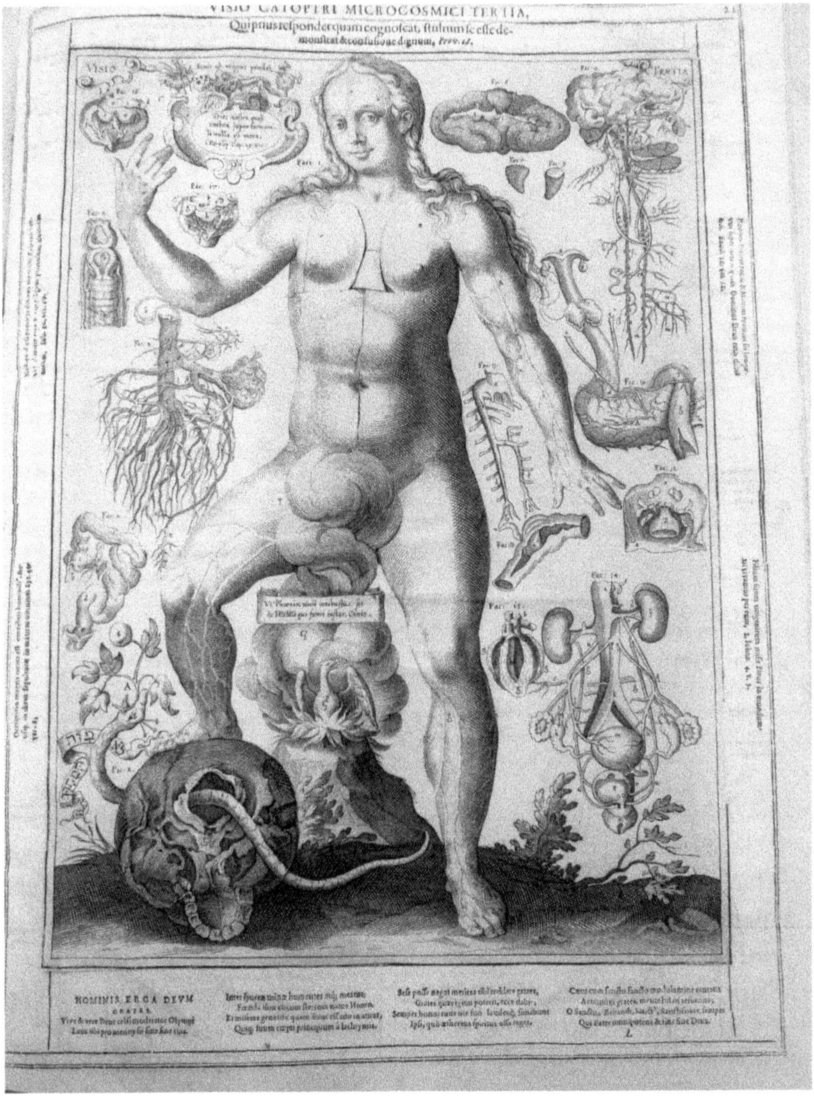

Figure 2.4. Johann Remmelin, 'Third Vision', 1619. Etching and engraving from *Catoptrum microcosmicum*. Wellcome Library, London. Photograph: Rosemary Moore.

outside, divine ethereality/monstrous embodiment.[5] These oppositions are clearly legible on the surface of the 'First Vision' where man and woman turn to face one another across the page. Even the body's internal organs are artfully arranged to suggest a synonymy based on morphological form,

5 Ibid.

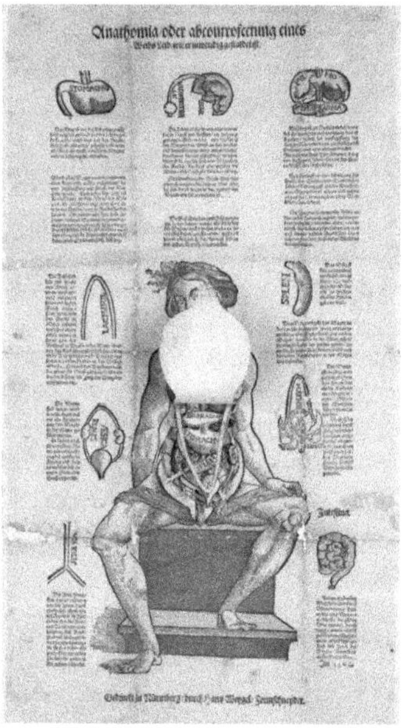

Figure 2.5. Jacob Frölich, after Heinrich Vogtherr, *Anatomy, or, a Faithful Reproduction of the Body of a Female*, 1544. Woodcut. 55 x 25 cm. Wellcome Library, London. Photograph: Wellcome Library.

while the aforementioned monstrous creature in the lower portion of the print is counterposed with a heavenly apparition above it. These oppositions will be explored in greater depth subsequently, but it is important to point out that arguments hinging on *surface appearances* overlook a key aspect of the print's design – its layering of highly complex, multifaceted paper flaps.

Significantly, Remmelin's print is no ordinary anatomical illustration. The *Catoptrum microcosmicum* triptych belong to an innovative category of anatomical print known as the 'fugitive sheet'. First appearing on the print market in Strasbourg, Germany, around 1538 with Heinrich Vogtherr's pair of female and male prints, fugitive sheets utilize paper flaps, carefully cut and pasted over one another to produce an approximation of three-dimensionality and interior space within the body or organ depicted (fig. 2.5).[6]

This clever use of cut-out components and layering conveys a sense of spatiality for the body, thus solving a long-standing problem for anatomical

6 For further information on the development and proliferation of the fugitive sheet, see Carlino, 'Paper Bodies'; Moore, 'Paper Cuts'.

illustration. But while the insertion of layers enables viewers to adopt a more active role than is usually presumed, this has both advantages and drawbacks for the prints. One downside is that many prints sustained irrevocable damage and were essentially 'thumbed out of existence'. They were either damaged beyond repair as a result of continued use, or pasted onto walls and furniture and subsequently lost. Some, however, were carefully stored away, folded between the pages of books, and for these surviving prints fingerprint stains, curling edges and little tears provide insight into how they may have been used.

Typically, when one encounters fugitive sheets in museums or galleries today, they are preserved under a protective layer of glass preventing one from touching them. Yet this could not be more different from how they were designed to be used. The delicate paper flaps are intended to be lifted, to allow users to peer *inside* the paper body and, in doing so, to bring new information into visibility through *hands-on* investigation. Of course, all prints have a unique connection with the bodies of those who use them. They are designed to be handled, not just looked at. They can be touched, coloured and adorned. Every surviving example of early modern prints therefore bears evidence of the wear and tear it has suffered in the hands of its users. However, for some prints more than others the user's intervention is more obvious and has more immediate effects on the visual image. This is the case for fugitive sheets, which attempt to meet the demand for bodies to be represented as 'naturally' as possible, at the same time as transforming the body into knowledge without abstracting its form.

Users engaged with and marked their prints in very different ways. Some even bear evidence of a ritualistic or talismanic belief in a print's perceived ability to shape or influence the present. For example, Suzanne Karr Schmidt draws attention to the traces of what appears to be blood, or an approximation of it, smeared on the genital region of a female anatomical print.[7] This raises the possibility of previously unconsidered uses for fugitive sheets. It is well known that wooden anatomical models were used for instructing women and young married couples about the reproductive process. Talismanic properties were also attributed to domestic objects like birth trays. These examples reveal how images were often invested with special significance and sometimes thought to have the power to influence the outcome of a pregnancy. Might fugitive sheets have held a similar function for some of their users?

7 Schmidt, *Altered and Adorned*, p. 91.

Undoubtedly the uses of fugitive prints are much more diverse than is usually presumed. It is no longer supposed that they were only of interest to specialist groups such as barber-surgeons, who could not read the classical anatomical texts in Latin but were required to have some knowledge of the human anatomy because they had the task of cutting the body during the public anatomy lessons held at universities.[8] It is now accepted that anatomical prints, including fugitive sheets, were used by a wide range of people and in diverse places.[9] Evidence even suggests that Remmelin's sheets may have been used to decorate the walls of anatomical theatres such as that at the University of Leiden.[10] Even so, the very success of the fugitive print has resulted in it being relegated to the category of 'popular' print. This is a problematic category, particularly since it assumes that the prints' appeal, though evidently far-reaching, was due to the moralistic premise that to know one's own anatomy was to contemplate the divine ingenuity of God. Of course, medicine and religious belief cannot be separated from one another, especially since the soul was frequently imagined as a physical part of the body. But the prints do not only address the soul, they also offer information about the physical concerns of ordinary people and provide information about illnesses and remedies.[11] These are highly complex objects, engaging with users on a number of levels and commenting on medical knowledge of the body, gendered identity, social status and religious doctrine. As Roger Chartier writes: 'By reintroducing variation and difference where the illusion of universality spontaneously springs up, such reflection may help us to get rid of some of our over sure distinctions and some over sure truisms.'[12]

Within the category of fugitive sheets, the *Catoptrum microcosmicum* triptych is often characterized as an outlier. For Lyle Massey, the prints can be 'distinguished from other flap sheets for the way they fabricate recondite associations between dissection and alchemy, and for their multiple inscriptions in Latin, Hebrew and Greek'.[13] Yet the use of images with moving parts has long been affiliated with the production of *different kinds* of knowledge. Fugitive sheets were not the first images designed to be cut out and assembled

8 Choulant, *History*, p. 156.

9 See Carlino, 'Paper Bodies', pp. 3, 104-113.

10 Huisman, *The Finger of God*, pp. 38-48.

11 For example, the fugitive sheet held in the Wellcome Library, *Interiorum corporis humani*, which is sometimes attributed to Thomas Geminus, represents the 'principal vaynes wvith the vse / of letting bludde' on the male figure while a separate sheet of text describes, in detail, the development of the fetus

12 Chartier, *The Order of Books*, p. xi.

13 Massey, 'The Alchemical Womb', p. 209.

by their users. Even earlier examples of experiments with moving parts are the devices known as volvelles. These are comprised of paper discs that can be layered on top of one another and sewn or glued onto the page so that they freely rotate around a central pivot. Volvelles were employed for many different purposes: medical charts, mystical divinations and astronomical instruments expedient as navigational aids. And crucially, they were always conceived of as a way of *producing*, not just conveying information.[14] This is a significant distinction and, though it is the case with all anatomical prints, has particular implications for fugitive sheets, which on occasion are associated with astrology and the divination of prophetic knowledge. Remmelin's 'First Vision' is a case in point since it represents human anatomy in combination with allegorical, philosophical and even occult forms of knowledge.

Technical innovations also distinguish the prints of the *Catoptrum microcosmicum* from earlier fugitive sheets. The problem, common to all extant sixteenth-century fugitive sheets, of rendering the body illegible as the user folds back the paper flaps is resolved in the 'First Vision' by printing the image on both sides. And removable parts allow users to extract some of the organs and inspect them more closely. In fact, some art historians point to the sheer complexity of their design as a means of differentiating them from the fugitive sheets printed in the sixteenth century.[15] In most fugitive sheets, all of the flaps are hinged in one place – the thorax – meaning that assemblies, while often imperfect or divergent, could nonetheless be carried out by untrained hands. The *Catoptrum microcosmicum* triptych has a far more complicated arrangement: some flaps can be lifted upwards, others can be pulled downwards or even folded outwards. This has led to speculation that the prints must have been pieced together by a specialist team of workers who had a guide – perhaps a preassembled manikin – to work from, potentially making them more costly than other fugitive sheets.[16] Though it seems unlikely that the prints were assembled after purchase by users, this does not rule out the possibilities of misuse, misappropriation and reshaping of the prints. Many copies of the triptych have had pigment applied by hand, all bear evidence of use through damage to the paper flaps and some even appear to have been intentionally defaced.

14 Amongst the earliest examples of volvelles are those attributed to Ramón Lull. See Lindberg, 'Mobiles in Books', p. 51.

15 Schmidt, *Altered and Adorned*, p. 85.

16 Ibid., p. 88. Massey points out that even this is speculative however, writing that 'its presumed costliness would seem to have relegated it to a highly select and elite audience, and yet its print history reveals prodigious editions in many languages'. See Massey, 'The Alchemical Womb', p. 209.

It is surprising, therefore, that much of the existing literature concerning the 'First Vision' overlooks the transient, interactive nature of the print's design, in favour of stressing the binary oppositions that exist at a surface level. In fact, as this chapter will explore, moving *under* the surface of the print one encounters a number of unexpected revelations that threaten the apparent stability of the symmetry and oppositions organizing its surface. My focus will be on the 'First Vision' only, although it is important to stress that the other two prints in the triptych likewise incorporate multifaceted, printed layers carefully arranged to mimic the spatiality of the body, organ or allegorical symbol represented. The fact that the materiality of the 'First Vision' threatens the clearly defined organizing principle suggested by the triptych's title and reiterated by much of the secondary literature is the central premise of this chapter. Instead of clear binary oppositions, I argue that the print – and thus the knowledge it seeks to reproduce – is actually far less stable than tends to be assumed. The varied implications of juxtaposing the pregnant female body with the 'monster' that partially obscures it are, I argue, representative of precisely this lack of stability and openness to interpretation. Like the maternal imagination – which was seen on the one hand to be perilous and corrupting, but also, conversely, as a means by which early modern men and women sought to control and positively influence the outcome of a pregnancy – there are multiple, often contradictory potentials that can be activated by the print's users. Might the slippery, ambiguous nature of the maternal imagination offer an alternative theoretical framework for understanding the conflation of allegorical, religious and medical imagery in the 'First Vision'? One that replaces rigid dichotomies with multiplicities of meanings, ambivalences and (mis)interpretations more in keeping with the interactive nature of the fugitive sheet?

Surface vs spatiality

In order to understand the conflict between surface and spatiality, it is necessary to start with the outermost layer of the 'First Vision'. As I have already suggested, there is a strong symmetry, perhaps even a hierarchy, in terms of the organization of the main figures, the accessory organs and the allegories that are found at this outermost level. At the top of the print, *manicules* draw attention inwards, towards a huge disembodied eye and an ear. Between these is a heavenly apparition; two angels, both dressed in fine robes, hold aloft a floral wreath. A sword and martyr's palm are tied together in the centre of the garland and the words of Sanctus, from the Eucharistic liturgy, form a

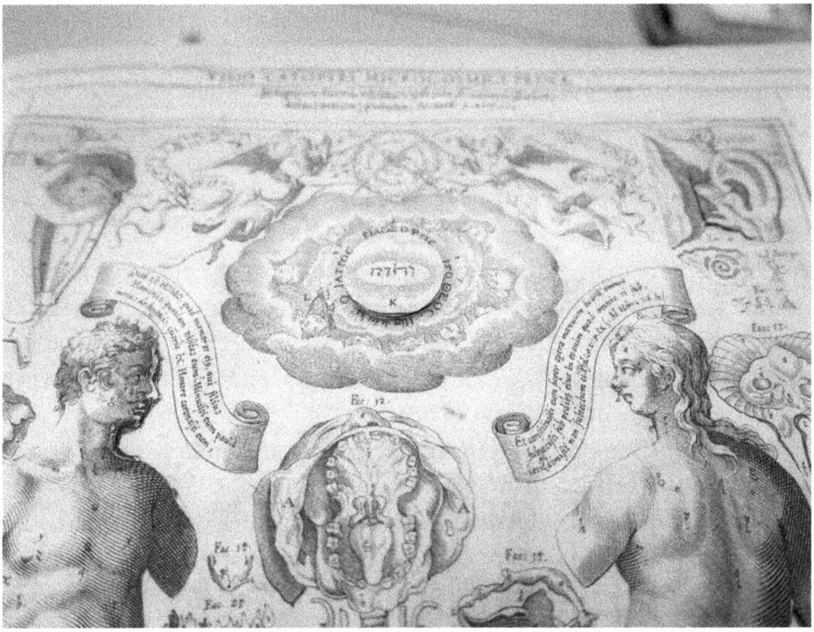

Figure 2.6. Detail of the Tetragrammaton in Johann Remmelin, 'First Vision', 1619. Etching and engraving from *Catoptrum microcosmicum*. Wellcome Library, London. Photograph: Rosemary Moore.

ring.[17] Beneath this, surrounded by a host of winged faces, one finds a cloud encircled Tetragrammaton, the Hebrew symbol for God usually transliterated as 'Yahweh'. Appropriately, many of the putti face inwards towards the word of God, but a few lift their little faces upwards to meet the viewer's gaze. With their mouths wide open as if in song, it is tempting to imagine these putti reciting the words of Psalm 34:8, which is printed around them: 'Oh taste and see that the Lord is good.'[18] This forms an intriguing counterpart to the 'monster' found emblazoned on the female torso at the bottom of the print. The serpent-haired creature also has its mouth wide open. However, it seems more likely to be emitting a tortured groan than chanting beatific verse. This point of comparison nonetheless serves to highlight the striking visual contrast between the celestial cloud above and the monstrous head below.

Elsewhere, the symmetry continues: a diminutive king's sceptre and a sexton's shovel mirror one another in terms of their verticality, even the internal organs – severed from their bodily context and distributed across

17 The words are: *Sanctus, Sanctus, Sanctus, Deus Zebaoth.*

18 This is written in Hebrew characters on the 1619 edition of the print. Significantly though, the Psalm is absent from the earlier 1613 edition of the 'First Vision'.

the printed page – are all aligned to complement and reflect one another. The figure labelled 'Facies 11', representing a membranous tissue known as the mesentery, and 'Facies 13', the diaphragm, perhaps best encapsulate the correspondence between the internal bodily parts. Although they have very different functions within the body, their shape and outline share a strong visual resemblance and for this reason the two are aligned, roughly level with one another, on opposite sides of the print. Moreover, as if to further accentuate how an invisible line of symmetry bisects the print, the limbless decapitated torso in the bottom centre has a cut running straight down the middle of its swollen belly. The triptych's title even draws on the metaphor of the mirror, though this was a well-known convention of late-sixteenth and early-seventeenth-century publications.[19] So too was the idea, stemming from ancient Greek philosophy, that the body of man acted as a kind of microcosm or 'little world' that mirrored the universe.

As a consequence of this striking symmetry, much of the scholarly literature focuses on the surface of the 'First Vision' – on the reflections and oppositions that, it is argued, are strategic to instilling order and therefore producing meaning for the print. And it is the antonymy between the 'monster' obscuring the genital region of the pregnant female torso and the heavenly apparition found at the top centre of the print that has attracted the most attention (figs 2.1, 2.6). These, it is argued, belong to a carefully devised schema conceived in terms of oppositions (male/female, part/whole, sacred/profane) that holds the threat of representational collapse at bay.[20] Yet the print's relation to the mirror metaphor is complex and problematic. On the one hand, the careful, deliberate placement of organs, allegories and texts produces the effect of balance. On the other hand, the insertion of layers *underneath* the print's surface, which are made visible by lifting an incision in the top layer, disrupts that carefully orchestrated order. As users penetrate beneath the surface of the print, meanings shift, new symmetries obscure old ones, and cracks in the mirror metaphor are revealed.

Interestingly, interpretations of the monstrous creature differ. Some claim it represents the devil, others describe it as Medusa's head. Yet, most agree that it is used to define the female body (and knowledge of it) as something unruly, potentially even dangerous or corrupting.[21] As Hillman and Mazzio

19 Grabes, *The Mutable Glass*, pp. 32-33.

20 Hillman and Mazzio, *The Body in Parts*, p. xvii.

21 Traub, 'Gendering Mortality', p. 84. Traub explains how it was a commonplace convention in late medieval and early modern visual culture to cover the male and female genitalia with an image of this kind. See also Massey, 'The Alchemical Womb', p. 219. Massey interprets Medusa's

write, 'the "unnameable" body part always potentially threatens the symbolic order of the Name of the Father, the order of meaning itself.'[22] Kate Cregan notes how the inscription of the words '*invidia* (envy), *orge* (anger), *neanias* (a young man or wilfulness), and *diabole* (slander)' on and around the monstrous head could denote four of the seven deadly sins of Christianity.[23] This, she concludes, makes an explicit connection between women's sexual organs and death by conveying the message that while the female body is the 'gate to terrestrial life' it is also potentially the gateway to 'eternal damnation'.[24] Massey writes: 'Secreting a woman's reproductive organs behind a devil's head, the *Catoptrum* regressively underlines Eve's/woman's association with initiating and participating in sin.'[25] Valerie Traub adopts a similar argument when she concludes that the head serves to equate the female body with sin and transgression by fixing woman's body as: 'the mortal site of primal sin and worldly knowledge'.[26] This is in pronounced contrast to the word of God directly above it, which can be seen as offering direct access to spiritual knowing and therefore to salvation. The assumption in all cases is that the monstrous head was appropriated by Remmelin for Christian moralizing purposes and that it only takes on meaning through its contrast with the Tetragrammaton.

However, lifting the outer layers of the print reveals that these oppositions are less stable than they initially appear. Provocatively, the print's users are invited to dissect the very word that defines God. Lifting the first layer of the Tetragrammaton reveals an etching of a plump cherub in keeping with the heavenly apparition that preceded it. The next layer represents an older, bearded man garbed in a bishop's mitre and fine robes.[27] The final layer is by far the most surprising of all. Buried deep beneath the Tetragrammaton, heavenly apparitions are substituted with a nightmarish impression of the devil's face (fig. 2.7).[28] At this point the apparent balance of oppositions

head as a devil's head but adopts a different approach to that of Traub, based on Remmelin and Michelspacher's known interest in alchemical knowledge and Paraclesian concepts of disease.

22 Hillman and Mazzio, *The Body in Parts*, p. xvii.

23 Cregan, 'Bodies', pp. 113-114. Cregan suggests their association with the sins of envy, wrath, pride and avarice.

24 Ibid., pp. 113-114.

25 Massey, 'The Alchemical Womb', p. 221.

26 Traub, 'Gendering Mortality', p. 84.

27 Massey suggests the identification of Hermes Trismegistus, which would make it an explicit link between anatomical knowledge and the ancient spiritual, mystical tradition of Hermeticism. Massey, 'The Alchemical Womb', p. 221.

28 In some copies this final image is absent. A Latin inscription is sometimes substituted in its place or added in as an additional layer. For further information, see Massey, 'The Alchemical Womb', p. 221.

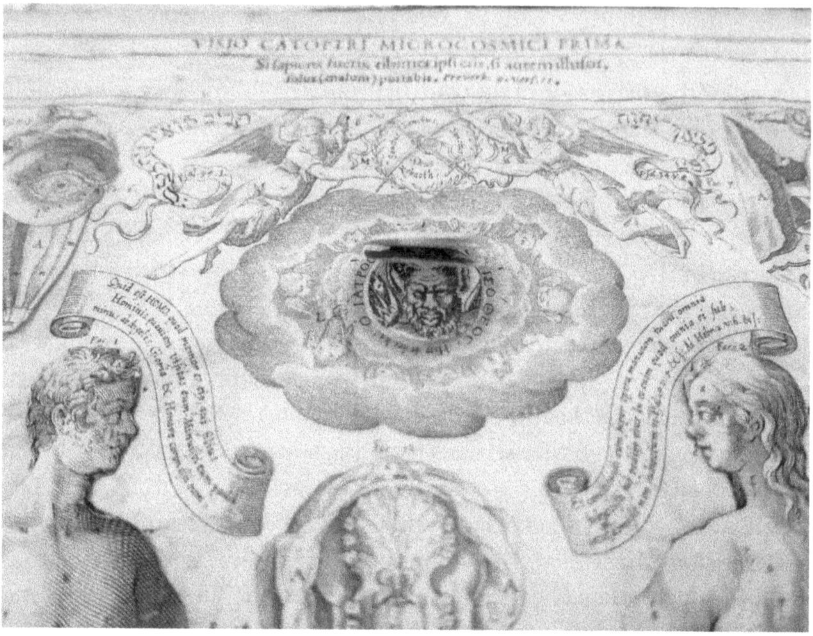

Figure 2.7. Detail of the devil in Johann Remmelin, 'First Vision', 1619. Etching and engraving from *Catoptrum microcosmicum*. Wellcome Library, London. Photograph: Rosemary Moore.

between godliness and monstrousness can no longer be argued to function. After all, how can the Tetragrammaton really claim to counter the monstrous head directly beneath it if an image of the devil can be found concealed between its layers?

Lifting the layers found underneath the monstrous head produces a similarly disconcerting effect. The first flap exposes the pudenda. This can be pulled downwards, and the abdomen opened outwards like the doors of a diptych, to reveal the internal anatomy of the womb. Delving deeper still into woman's body, one eventually arrives at a tiny fetus curled up inside its mother's womb (fig. 2.8). This too is printed onto a moveable flap. In fact, it is the final flap in this area of the print. Gently folding it downwards produces the impression that one is acting out its birth, as it takes the unborn child out of view and leaves one contemplating the now empty uterus. These multiple, shifting visions produced through the layering of the print certainly complicate the idea of a straightforward binary opposition. But even were it not for the insertion of layers in the print, the surface of the 'First Vision' reveals itself to be far from stable. Indeed, it is this instability that I will turn to address next.

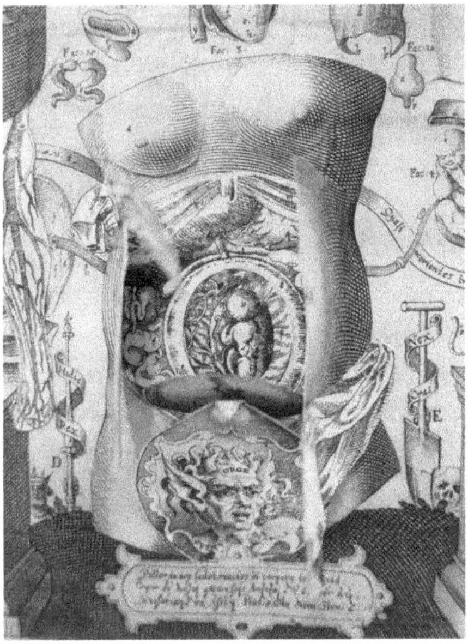

Figure 2.8. Detail of the fetus in Johann Remmelin, 'First Vision', 1619. Etching and engraving from *Catoptrum microcosmicum*. Wellcome Library, London. Photograph: Rosemary Moore.

An unstable surface

At this point, it is important to clarify that my analysis is based on the 1619 edition of the *Catoptrum microcosmicum* held in the Wellcome Library in London.[29] Amongst the few known surviving copies of the triptych dispersed across various collections no two are exactly alike. The technology of print might have allowed for an element of multiple copies to be produced but these objects were still pieced together by hand, meaning each one has variations. Over time, parts have been lost or damaged, and, in some cases, they may even have been intentionally destroyed or defaced. Each copy of the print exists in a different state due to the intervention of users and the damage and transformations that occurred over time.

To complicate matters further, multiple editions of the triptych were in circulation from the time it first appeared anonymously on the print market in 1613, to the last known restrikes of those plates published in Verona by a

29 Remmelin, *Catoptrum microcosmicum*, held in the Wellcome Library, London.

book dealer in 1754.[30] Writing in the preface to the first 'authorized' edition of 1619, Remmelin claimed that it had never been his intention to publish the prints. He even describes his surprise at having learnt of their entering onto the print market without his prior consent:

> [B]ut it so happened that the general talk of it among his friends caused the work to be wrested away from him for inspection and circulation, until, through their persuasion and at their expense, it began to be published, without his knowledge, and so to be enjoyed like an unripe fruit; but when he discovered that it abounded in defects, and teemed with numerous intolerable errors made by the engraver and printer, he again, albeit unwillingly, took up the work which he had designed 14 years earlier, revised it, and thus offered it in another dress.[31]

Despite Remmelin's protestations, it was common for authors to withhold their names from a publication until the second edition, when its success had been proven.[32] Moreover, very few alterations were actually made to the anatomical content of the prints. It was the moralistic and allegorical inscriptions – the focus of much scholarly attention – that saw the most dramatic changes. The psalms inscribed on the banderoles, the little allegorical scenes inside the roundels on the marble plinths, the king clutching his sceptre and the skull beside the shovel were all new additions to the 1619 edition. The fact that the monstrous head and the Tetragrammaton predate these implies that the author/printer recognized these two features alone do not produce the kind of stable, moralistic message that is often assumed. They thus remain paradoxically persistent, yet difficult to pin down.

As a consequence of its placement on a delicate paper flap on the outermost of the print's layers, the monstrous head is absent from a number of editions of the 'First Vision'.[33] Surely if it is intended to fix meanings, it would be secured on an area of the print less susceptible to damage or

30 The 1754 edition was published under the title: *Archangeli Piccolomini Anatome integra, revisa, tabulis explanata et iconibus mirificam humani corporis fabricam, ad ipsum naturae archetypum exprimentibus, cum preafatione et emendation Joann. Fantoni, Veronae, sumptib. Gabrielis Julii de Ferrariis*. It was misleadingly claimed by the book dealer to be the work of the anatomist Piccolhomini. For further information, see Choulant, *History*, p. 233.

31 Translation of Remmelin's text as given in McDaniel, 'The Affair', p. 433.

32 Ibid.

33 For example, the 1613 copy of the *Catoptrum microcosmicum* held at the Art Institute of Chicago has no flaps at all covering the genitals of the female torso. For a detailed discussion of this particular copy of Remmelin's prints, see Schmidt, *Altered and Adorned*, pp. 82-92, 101-104.

removal. These ambiguities are only confounded by the fact that its identification is also elusive. Though sometimes labelled a devil, the creature also shares characteristics of the mythological gorgon, Medusa. In addition to the hair being comprised of a mass of writhing, coiling snakes, the Latin inscription directly beneath it is taken from a passage in Book II of Ovid's *Metamorphoses:* 'Pallor spreads over her face, and all her body shrivels.'[34] While not directly related to the myth of Medusa, the text is nonetheless concerned with envious women and the power to transform flesh into stone, suggesting a strong link with the mythological gorgon.[35]

I would like to propose one possible interpretation of the monstrous head. *If* it is read as Medusa, then it raises questions about vision and the *productive* – not just destructive – potentials of the gorgon's severed head in the 'First Vision'. After all, one glimpse of Medusa is said to turn her victims into stone. But once cut, Medusa's head is, according to legend, transformed into an emblem of knowledge and power. First, it is utilized by the hero Perseus who holds it up to turn his enemies to stone, then later Athena, the goddess of wisdom and warfare, fixes it to her aegis.[36] Much like the way the anatomist's cuts work on the dead body, Perseus's cut therefore transforms Medusa's head from something monstrous – an object of fear and disgust – into an emblem of knowledge and power. Even more significantly, in Ovid's *Metamorphoses* the moment Perseus decapitates the gorgon her spilt blood gives rise to new life. As the following extract describes, Perseus '[s]evered the head, and from that mother's bleeding / Were born the swift-winged Pegasus and his brother.'[37] This is significant because the cut does not simply neutralize Medusa's threat by killing her, it also presents a portal through which new life is generated. As Tove Paulsson Holmberg argues, such affinity between birth, suffering and death was a persistent feature of early modern discourse on the labour of birth.[38] It is intriguing, however, that in this case labour is transferred from the gorgon Medusa to the hero Perseus, who brings Pegasus and Chrysaor into being by his sword, much as the anatomist generates knowledge by his scalpel, or the user of the print by their re-enactment of the cut.

34 The Latin inscription reads: *Pallor in ore sedet, macies in corpore toto*. Ovid, *Metamorphoses* (Miller), p. 114.

35 The second inscription, written in Greek, also alludes to the envious nature of women. The line is taken from Pindar's *Nemean Ode* 8 and translated reads: 'Words are a dainty morsel for the envious; and envy always clings to the noble, and has no quarrel with worse men.' Translation as given in Massey, 'The Alchemical Womb', p. 225.

36 Garber and Vickers, 'Introduction', p. 4.

37 Ovid, *Metamorphoses* (Humphries), p. 106.

38 Paulsson Holmberg, 'Ambiguous and Transitional Bodies', in this volume.

Monsters and the maternal

The ambiguous, even contradictory, nature of Medusa's head makes it comparable with early modern notions of the 'maternal imagination', which was, on the one hand, a potentially corrupting influence to be feared, whilst, on the other, an opportunity for control over an unborn child's development. The widely held belief that the female imagination – especially a woman's fears and desires – had the power to shape and ultimately distort the natural formation of an unborn child had its roots in antiquity. Yet it persisted up to the beginning of the nineteenth century.[39] References to the phenomena of 'visual imprinting' are commonplace in early modern texts. The influential protestant reformist Martin Luther spoke about a woman who gave birth to a mouse after one surprised her during pregnancy; the humanist scholar, Benedetto Varchi, likewise cited maternal imagination as one of the main causes of monstrous births; while the eminent Parisian surgeon Ambroise Paré wrote a whole chapter on the subject in his medical treatise of 1575.[40] But visual imprinting worked both ways: if the sight of something horrifying resulted in monstrous births, then it followed that gazing on images of perfectly healthy, chubby, male babies must have a positive impact. Art historians, including Jacqueline Marie Musacchio and Frances Gage, have contributed much to understandings of how this seemingly contradictory aspect of the maternal imagination manifested itself in the visual culture of the period, especially in the form of paintings and sculpture thought to have the ability to alter the appearance of an unborn child through visual imprinting.[41] This belief in the power of 'sympathetic magic' offers insight into why, in fifteenth- and sixteenth-century Italy, patrician families commissioned birth trays, adorned with images of plump, naked, *male* children. By contemplating what were considered by the society that produced them to be 'ideal' models, the hope was that the unruly maternal imagination might be tamed – or at least kept under some degree of control – thereby limiting the chances of so-called 'monstrous births'. It is also why pregnant women were given gifts of coral, a material believed to be imbued with special apotropaic powers. These same protective qualities of coral are associated with the myth of Medusa: blood from her freshly severed head drips into the ocean, falling onto the soft stems of seaweed, petrifying them.

39 Ovid, *Metamorphoses* (Humphries), p. 1.

40 Musacchio, *Art and Ritual*, p. 128. See also Paré, *On Monsters*.

41 Musacchio, *Art and Ritual*; Gage, *Painting*.

Like the maternal imagination, Medusa's head is also highly ambiguous by nature. Various suggestions abound as to why Medusa might be positioned over the pregnant torso's genitals, but most attribute it to a kind of warning about the dangers of seeing too much.[42] Nonetheless, it remains unclear as to whether Medusa's head is intended to protect the male viewer against the dangers of confronting the potentially corrupting female body, as it was in the myth of Perseus and the gorgon, or to protect the female body from the penetrating male gaze. Hillman and Mazzio even comment on the remarkable way in which it seems to prefigure the influential analysis of Medusa's head as a castration symbol in Sigmund Freud's essay 'Medusa's Head', written in 1922 and published posthumously in 1940.[43] Freud succinctly encapsulated his analysis in the equation 'To decapitate = to castrate'.[44] The analysis is based around a fear of castration, yet Freud wrote that Medusa's head also contained the possibility of mitigating that horror since the coiled snakes of her hair could be read as multiple phalluses, transforming her into a reassuring penis symbol. Traub describes the Medusa's head in Remmelin's print in a similar way to Freud when she writes that it is intended to compensate for the male viewer's 'dread of the female genital interior'.[45]

Another interpretation is that Medusa's head is merely intended to obfuscate the female genitals, hence preserving male desire by not showing too much.[46] This relegates it to the same function as the illusionistic fabric ties layered over the breasts and around the hips to prevent the 'doors' of the torso's belly from curling upwards and prematurely bringing the 'secrets of women' into visibility.[47] Yet, this strategy would be fundamentally flawed because far from concealing the female sexual organs, Medusa suggestively evokes the opening of the vagina. As Cregan points out, the outline of the flap into which Medusa's head is printed follows the contours of the labia majora, the inner tracery can be likened to the labia minora, and the teardrop shape inscribed with the word *invidia* could be seen as the clitoris. The open mouth can even be compared with the vaginal opening.[48] In effect, it replicates what it hides.

Even more intriguingly, the tapered top of the flap bearing Medusa's head points towards a perpendicular incision that runs straight down the centre

42 Hillman and Mazzio, *The Body in Parts*, p. xvii; Cregan, 'Bodies', p. 113; Traub, *The Renaissance*, p. 122; Eggert, *Disknowledge*, p. 178.

43 Freud, 'Medusa's Head', pp. 273-275.

44 Ibid., p. 273.

45 Traub, *The Renaissance*, p. 122.

46 Eggert, *Disknowledge*, p. 178.

47 I borrow the phrase from Park, *Secrets of Women*.

48 Cregan, 'Bodies', p. 114.

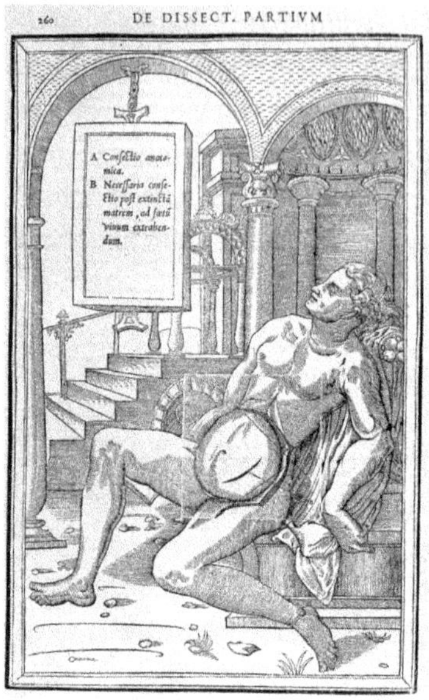

Figure 2.9. Charles Estienne, Female anatomical model showing the location of the caesarean cut, 1545. Woodcut from p. 260 of Charles Estienne, *De dissectione partium corporis humani* [On the dissection of the parts of the human body] (Parisiis: Apud Simonem Colinaeum, 1545). Photograph: Wellcome Library.

of the pregnant torso's belly, splitting the umbilicus in two. This in turn recalls the kind of precise, surgical cut that would have been performed in a caesarean operation. However, as a woodcut for Book II of Charles Estienne's *De dissectione partium corporis humani* [On the dissection of the parts of the human body] (1545) makes evident, the mother was unlikely to survive the operation (fig. 2.9).[49]

A caesarean also features in Ovid's *Metamorphoses* when Apollo surgically extracts his son Asclepius, god of medicine, from the abdomen of the mortal Coronis. It is fitting, then, that Medusa should be aligned with the caesarean cut since in some versions of the myth blood from her sides is

49 The procedure was more commonly known as a caesarean operation up until the end of the sixteenth century. The term 'caesarean section' seems to have been first introduced by Jacques Guillemeau, though he advised against the operation except as a post-mortem procedure. For the English translation, see Guillemeau, *The Happy Delivery of Women*. See the woodcut in Estienne, *De dissectione partium corporis humani*.

said to have been given to Asclepius. According to the legend: 'That drawn from the left [possessed] the power to raise the dead, while that from the right could destroy whoever drank it.'[50] Lisa Rosenthal describes how the power of Medusa's head is intrinsically linked to these ambiguities stemming from the fact it has both deadly and procreative potency.[51] Similarly to how Medusa's spilled blood spawned two offspring in the form of Pegasus the winged horse and Chrysaor the giant, two offspring are also resultant of the caesarean incision in Remmelin's print. On either side of the truncated torso billowing banderoles spiral outwards, like spurts of blood. These recall the ribbon-like streams of blood-red pigment that issue forth from Medusa's severed neck in Caravaggio's painting of c. 1570/1610, *Medusa* (Uffizi Gallery, Florence), which depicts the precise moment the head is cut from the body. Remmelin's print, however, represents Medusa at the moment the cut remakes her head as something new – something productive. And from her spilled blood, represented by the banderoles, the main male and female anatomical models appear to materialize. Their missing limbs have not yet fully formed. The process of materialization is not yet complete in the 'First Vision'. But the two offspring will step down from their stone plinths, fully formed, to become the central focus of the second and third 'visions' of the triptych.

Ultimately, the spatialization of the print reveals how apparent oppositions are not as clear cut as they initially appear. Through interactions with the print, users bring new aspects into visibility, thereby obscuring or problematizing existing ones. Crucially, this lack of fixity, this susceptibility to outside influences, makes the print comparable to how the pregnant female body and the maternal imagination were conceptualized during the seventeenth century. Like the maternal imagination, the monster/Medusa evokes the dangerous and unruly aspect of the female anatomy, but, as I hope to have shown, it also suggests its *productive* nature. It gives rise to new life forms and can even be used as a protective, apotropaic device. Indeed, it is precisely this multifaceted, ambiguous nature of Remmelin's 'First Vision' that makes the maternal imagination such a useful analytic tool for thinking through some of its possibilities. Whilst I have suggested one possible alternative interpretation of the monstrous head that haunts the lower region of the 'First Vision', this is by no means the only possible reading. Rather, I hope that this might begin to open up a dialogue about the multiplicities of meanings that can be found just below the surface of

50 Sawday, *The Body Emblazoned*, p. 9.
51 Rosenthal, *Gender, Politics*, p. 182.

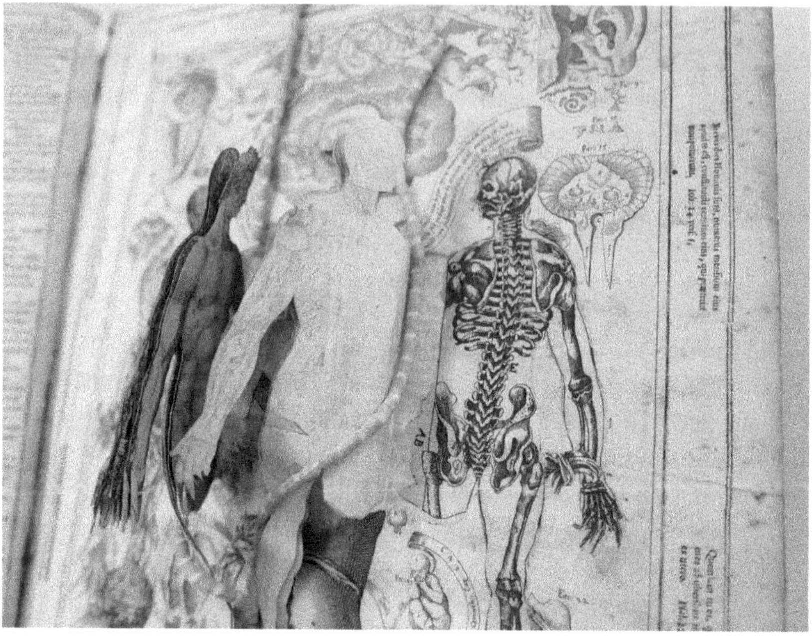

Figure 2.10. Detail of the main anatomical figures with the flaps raised. From Johann Remmelin, 'First Vision', 1619. Etching and engraving from *Catoptrum microcosmicum*. Wellcome Library, London. Photograph: Rosemary Moore.

Remmelin's print, and of its many possible uses, misuses and (mis)interpretations at the hands of different users.

Finally, even as the user's intervention disrupts the binaries of good/evil, divine/corrupting, male/female by spatializing the print, a new form of symmetry emerges as users dissect the paper bodies on display. Lifting the layers of the two main anatomical figures has unexpected consequences. All of the flaps hinge on one side of the body – the side closest to the centre of the print – with the result that as one turns them over a new kind of symmetry is produced. The figures' faces are represented in profile so the overturned flaps form a mirror image that stares back at the body they are derived from – in effect, they scrutinize one another. And, though the verso of the flap is not printed with any anatomical features, the faint outline of features on the recto, including the face, the contours of musculature – even the fig leaf concealing Adam's genitals – are *just* visible through the thin, porous paper. It is as if the figures have turned their attention away from the outward appearance of things, in order to look *inside themselves*. One could argue that, as a consequence of this, the focus of the print is reorientated so that the two anatomical figures, not the Tetragrammaton and the monstrous head, become the new locus of symmetry within the 'First Vision'. But unlike the symmetry of the mirror, the multiple layers contained with the body not only reflect the body, they replicate it over and over again – and each time it adopts a slightly different form.

Works Cited

Carlino, Andrea, 'Paper Bodies: A Catalogue of Anatomical Fugitive Sheets, 1538-1687', *Medical History. Supplement* 19 (1999), pp. 1-352.

Chartier, Roger, *The Order of Books: Readers, Authors, and Libraries in Europe between the Fourteenth and Eighteenth Centuries*, trans. Lydia G. Cochrane (Cambridge: Polity, 1994).

Choulant, Ludwig, *History and Bibliography of Anatomical Illustration*, trans. Frank Mortimer (Chicago: University of Chicago Press, 1920).

Cregan, Kate, 'Bodies Acted "To teach man wherein hee is imperfect"', in *The Theatre of the Body: Staging Death and Embodying Life in Early-Modern London* (Turnhout: Brepols, 2009), pp. 101-134.

Daston, Lorraine, and Katharine Park, *Wonders and the Order of Nature, 1150-1750* (New York: Zone Books, 1998).

Eggert, Katherine, *Disknowledge: Literature, Alchemy, and the End of Humanism in Renaissance England* (Philadelphia: University of Pennsylvania Press, 2015).

Estienne, Charles, *De dissectione partium corporis humani* [On the dissection of the parts of the human body] (Parisiis: Apud Simonem Colinaeum, 1545).

Freud, Sigmund, 'Medusa's Head (1940 [1922])', in *The Complete Psychological Works of Sigmund Freud, vol. 18: Beyond the Pleasure Principal, Group Psychology and Other Works (1920-1922)*, trans. James Strachey (London: Hogarth Press and The Institute of Psycho-Analysis, 1955), pp. 273-275.

Gage, Frances, *Painting as Medicine in Early Modern Rome: Giulio Mancini and the Efficacy of Art* (University Park: Pennsylvania State University Press, 2016).

Garber, Marjorie, and Nancy J. Vickers, 'Introduction', in *The Medusa Reader*, ed. Marjorie Garber and Nancy J. Vickers (New York: Routledge, 2003), pp. 1-9.

Grabes, Herbert, *The Mutable Glass: Mirror-Imagery in Titles and Texts of the Middle Ages and English Renaissance*, trans. Gordon Collier (Cambridge: Cambridge University Press, 1982).

Guillemeau, J., *The Happy Delivery of Women*, trans. A. Hatfield (London: A. Hatfield, 1612).

Hillman, David, and Carla Mazzio, 'Introduction: Individual Parts', in *The Body in Parts: Fantasies of Corporeality in Early Modern Europe*, ed. David Hillman and Carla Mazzio (New York: Routledge, 1997), pp. xi-xxiv.

Huet, Marie Hélène, *Monstrous Imagination* (Cambridge, MA: Harvard University Press, 1993).

Huisman, Tim, *The Finger of God: Anatomical Practice in 17th-Century Leiden* (Leiden: Primavera Pers, 2009).

Lindberg, Sten G., 'Mobiles in Books: Volvelles, Inserts, Pyramids, Divinations and Children's Games', *Private Library*, 3rd series, 2, no. 2 (1979), pp. 49-82.

Massey, Lyle, 'The Alchemical Womb: Johann Remmelin's *Catoptrum microcosmicum*', in *The Visual Culture of Secrecy*, ed. Timothy McCall, Sean Roberts and Giancarlo Fiorenza (Kirksville: Truman State University Press, 2013), pp. 208-229.

McDaniel, W.B., 'The Affair of the "1613" Printing of Johannes Rümelin's *Catoptron*', *Transactions and Studies of the College of Physicians of Philadelphia*, 4th series, 6 (1938), pp. 60-72.

Monogrammist R.S., *Interiorum corporis humani partium viva delineatio*, in *Compendiosa totius anatomie delineation* (London: Thomas Geminus, 1559).

Moore, Rosemary, 'Paper Cuts: The Early Modern Fugitive Print', *Object* 17 (2015), pp. 54-76.

Musacchio, Jacqueline Marie, *The Art and Ritual of Childbirth in Renaissance Italy* (New Haven: Yale University Press, 1999).

Ovid, *Metamorphoses*, trans. Rolfe Humphries (Bloomington: Indiana University Press, 1983).

Ovid, *Metamorphoses Books 1-8 with an English Translation by Frank Justus Miller*, trans. Frank Justus Miller, new ed. (Cambridge, MA: Harvard University Press, 2014).

Paré, Ambroise, *On Monsters and Marvels* (Chicago: University of Chicago Press, 1983).

Park, Katharine, *Secrets of Women: Gender, Generation, and the Origins of Human Dissection* (New York: Zone Books, 2006).

Remmelin, Johann, *Catoptrum microcosmicum* (Augsburg: Typis Davidis Francki, 1619).

Rosenthal, Lisa, *Gender, Politics, and Allegory in the Art of Rubens* (Cambridge: Cambridge University Press, 2005).

Sawday, Jonathan, *The Body Emblazoned: Dissection and the Human Body in Renaissance Culture* (London: Routledge, 1995).

Schmidt, Suzanne Karr, *Altered and Adorned: Using Renaissance Prints in Daily Life* (New Haven: Yale University Press, 2011).

Traub, Valerie, 'Gendering Mortality in Early Modern Anatomies', in *Feminist Readings of Early Modern Culture: Emerging Subjects*, ed. Valerie Traub, Lindsay M. Kaplan and Dympna Callaghan (Cambridge: Cambridge University Press, 1996), pp. 44-92.

Traub, Valerie, *The Renaissance of Lesbianism in Early Modern England* (Cambridge: Cambridge University Press, 2002).

About the Author

Rosemary Moore is Teaching Fellow in Early Modern European Art and Culture at University College London. She works on sixteenth- and seventeenth-century print culture, with a particular focus on the visual culture of medicine. Previous publications have examined how cutting altered and reshaped the relation between image and body in early modern anatomical prints.

3. The Optics of Bodily Deviance: Juan Ruiz de Alarcón's Path to Public Office[1]

Pablo García Piñar

Abstract
Through an account of New Spanish playwright Juan Ruiz de Alarcón y Mendoza's path to secure an administrative position for himself in seventeenth-century Spain's Hapsburg administrative apparatus, this essay discusses the cultural and social conditions that led to the administration's persistent preoccupation with its public image and, in particular, with the safeguarding of its authority. I argue that the instances of public contempt expressed by his peers – on account of the severe bodily deformity Ruiz de Alarcón suffered from – played a decisive role in the decision of the Council of the Indies to ban the playwright from any public office. The council's behaviour reflects the restraining influence that the Hapsburg administration exercised over the physical appearance of state officials. This essay also discusses how Ruiz de Alarcón challenges the logic behind this disciplining of bodily appearance in his play *Las paredes oyen*.

Keywords: history of state administration, authority, disability studies, deformity, bodily deviance, early modern Spanish theatre

On 1 July 1625, the secretary of the Council of the Indies issued a report regarding the fitness of New Spanish playwright Juan Ruiz de Alarcón y Mendoza for a permanent position in one of the Audiencias de las Indias,

1 I would like to express my deepest gratitude to my father, Antonio García Reche, a retired general practitioner, for helping me to understand and describe the extent of Ruiz de Alarcón's condition.

Bondestam, M. (ed.), *Exceptional Bodies in Early Modern Culture: Concepts of Monstrosity before the Advent of the Normal*. Taylor & Francis Group, 2020
DOI 10.5117/9789463721745_CH03

the appeals court system in the Spanish territories in the New World. King Phillip IV had entrusted the report to the council's president, Juan de Villela, and it was sent out as a response to a memorandum Ruiz de Alarcón had presented before the council. The document replicated the merits that the playwright listed in his memorandum: two bachelor's degrees awarded by the prestigious University of Salamanca – in Canon Law in 1600 and Civil Law in 1602 – and another degree in Civil Law from the University of Mexico received in 1609. Ruiz de Alarcón claimed, in addition, to have defended cases before the Royal Audience of Seville in 1607 and before the Royal Audience of Mexico from 1611 to 1612. Apart from his merits, the playwright reminded the council that neither his grandparents nor their descendants had received any reward for being among the first discoverers and settlers of the silver-mining region of Teotlalco, present day Taxco, in New Spain. In reality, enumerating his merits was a mere formality in order to justify his credentials: by 1625 Ruiz de Alarcón was not only one of the most successful playwrights of his age, but he also enjoyed the protection of Don Ramiro Núñez de Guzmán, son-in-law of the count-duke of Olivares – royal favourite of Philip IV and, at that moment, the most powerful man in the Spanish Empire. In spite of this seemingly advantageous position, Ruiz de Alarcón's efforts to secure a stable position for himself in the Spanish administrative apparatus had been, up until that moment, a path strewn with obstacles and disappointments.

Juan Ruiz de Alarcón was born before 30 December 1572, the date of his baptism in the Real de Minas de Tetelcuitlacinco, into a family dedicated to the extraction of silver – by then already declining. Apart from Ruiz de Alarcón's certificate of baptism, almost nothing is known about him before 1596, the year in which the playwright enrolled at the Royal and Pontifical University of Mexico, where he studied canon law until 1600. In May of the same year, he departed for the Iberian Peninsula in order to continue his studies at the University of Salamanca and, due to financial difficulties, he left his studies sometime around 1606 or 1607, and returned to Mexico City in 1608. Once there, even though he graduated *in utroque iure* – as a doctor on both civil and canon laws – on 21 February 1609, Ruiz de Alarcón never received his doctorate degree due to unknown reasons. On four occasions, from 1609 to 1613, he strove to attain a professor position in the law school. After his last attempt, on 30 April 1613, in which he competed against other four candidates for a chair in Roman civil law, Ruiz de Alarcón filed several complaints with the academic senate denouncing a number of irregularities in the process, including an extremely serious accusation: vote coercion.[2]

2 Rangel, 'Noticias biográficas', p. 23.

Following this final setback, probably aware that his protests had burned his bridges with the law school, Ruiz de Alarcón embarked for Spain once more on 21 May. He would never return again to the New World.

The report drawn up by the Council of the Indies favourably evaluated the merits that Ruiz de Alarcón had presented. In the document, Villela declared that the council had 'always been satisfied with his knowledge and was aware of his talents' ('*ha tenido siempre satisfacción de sus letras y conocido su talento*'). Despite the council's estimation that the playwright's aptitudes made him worthy of a position in the Audiencias Reales, they judged that he was not fit to fill a public position. The reason, explained Villela, was 'the bodily defect that he has, which is sizable for the authority required to represent such an office' ('*el defecto corporal que tiene, el cual es grande para la autoridad que ha menester representar en cosa semejante*').[3]

According to Villela's statement, it can be argued that the council felt that Ruiz de Alarcón's physical appearance – marked by a divergent bodily configuration, the particulars of which I will discuss below – could severely interfere with the deferential regard with which the Hapsburg administration intended each and every of its officials to be addressed. As I will argue here, while bodily deviations were rendered laughable, offensive and revolting, they were also considered to be a manifestation of underlying moral weaknesses and, therefore, a debilitating factor for the imposition of authority. The council's attitude, thus, betrays the central role that physical appearance played in what the Hapsburg administration regarded to be the legitimizing sources of authority. Ruiz de Alarcón's whole trajectory raises the question of what constituted a regular – or regular enough – body in the context of the Spanish state's administrative apparatus, and what constitutes an extraordinary body, one selected to be excluded from that apparatus.

The bad optics of unfit bodies

The concern with the adequation between the dignity of the position and its aesthetic realization in the body of the state official, I argue, can be considered as a by-product of the socio-economic and cultural conditions at play in the refoundation of the Spanish administrative system in the sixteenth century. The impetus with which Spain expanded its domains across the globe caused an urgent need in the state's administrative apparatus to enlarge its bureaucratic infrastructure. Since the former

3 Fernández-Guerra y Orbe, *Don Juan Ruiz de Alarcón*, p. 523.

recruitment pools the administration drew upon during the pre-Empire period – fundamentally law-trained nobility – were insufficient to satisfy the demands of the imperial project, the administrative apparatus began to massively absorb legally trained professionals coming from lower strata, such as the low nobility and the urban bourgeoisie.[4] Given the scale of the imperial project, traditional qualification methods were deemed obsolete by the state, which began to entrust the recruitment of new public servants to high-ranking state officials. Once the administration had gained control over the appointment of bureaucratic personnel, notes Richard Kagan, it began to recruit individuals with a profile similar to their own: the same social extraction and academic training.[5] This amalgamating process, argues José Antonio Maravall, did not only give shape to a new estate of the realm, but also generated a social group with a strong class-consciousness.[6] The caste of state officials soon developed its own distinctive group identity, characterized by the formation of its own social culture and the preoccupation with their position on the social scale – and, therefore, with the way they were perceived from the outside.

The above societal shift stimulated the newly formed estate – which was experiencing unprecedented prosperity – to permeate the social sphere of the hegemonic classes. In their lure for intermingling with the upper social classes, public officials began to cultivate the refined manners that would previously have been distinctive to the nobility. The preoccupation shown by the Hapsburg administration with bodily representation of authority probably had its origin in the popularity of courtesy handbooks, such as Baldassare Castiglione's *The Book of the Courtier* (1528) or Giovanni Della Casa's *Galateo* (1558), in which the concern about the individual's public image was central. Accounts of the desirable physical features that a public servant should embody can be found in the pages of a number of political treaties composed by authors involved in the state administration. For instance, just to name a few, *El concejo, y consejeros del príncipe* (1559), a book belonging to the genre of mirror for princes by Fadrique Furió Ceriol, counsellor of Philip II of Spain, devotes a whole section to determining which bodily features were advantageous for the image of the royal counsellor and which ones were detrimental. In his *Tractado del consejo y de los consejeros de los príncipes* (1584), Bartolomeu Filippe, professor of canon law at the University of Coimbra, advocates for the exclusion from public office of

4 Vincens Vives, *Coyuntura económica*, pp. 123-133; Maravall, *Estado moderno*, II, pp. 487-498.

5 Kagan, *Students*, p. 90.

6 Maravall, 'Los "hombres de saber"', II, pp. 361-362.

applicants with unattractive bodily attributes, while Jerónimo Castillo de Bobadilla, prosecutor of the Royal Chancery of Valladolid, argues in his *Política para corregidores y señores de vassallos* (1597) that a harmonious physical appearance would most easily persuade individuals to comply with authority. Unlike the extraordinary bodies depicted in collections of prodigies about a century later, such as Johannes Schefferus's 'Variae historiae' – which, as Maja Bondestam demonstrates,[7] were meant to elicit in the reader a reflection upon the inner workings of nature – the sections in these treaties devoted to the tabulation and discussion of objectionable bodily features were intended to provoke in the reader a distrust of those anatomical lineaments that deviated from what was considered desirable.

Even though the exact origins of this bodily aesthetic remain unclear, one could claim that its leading disseminator was the enormously influential *El concejo, y consejeros del príncipe*. *El concejo* was a fulgurant success all over the Old Continent: in a 60-year period, it was translated into four languages – Latin, Italian, English and Polish – in a total of ten separate editions, and it had a substantial influence on political thought in the Iberian Peninsula. While *El concejo* was extensively quoted in political treatises, most Spanish authors addressing the question of the state official's bodily appearance noticeably regarded him as the highest authority in the matter.

In *El concejo*, Furió Ceriol advised Phillip II on both the kind of education the prince should receive and how the upper echelons of the state apparatus should be organized. One of the fundamental discussions of this work focuses on the selection process of the councils that administered the empire. Furió Ceriol believed that an intellectual and moral elite, chosen by virtue of their merit and competence, should form the council. The counsellor that Furió Ceriol imagined should be a cultured and worldly man, a wise strategist in the political realm, who should be guided by cardinal and theological virtues. Along with intellectual, political, and moral skills, this ideal advisor should also fit an anatomical canon, determined as much by age as by temperament, physical size and bodily proportion. In accordance with the parameters that Furió Ceriol deemed appropriate, the counsellor should be 'of average shape in height and weight; because any excess in this matter seems bad and takes away the authority pertaining to the counsellor'.[8] In effect, the ideal counsellor should be of moderate height, because, if excessively tall, 'they do not hesitate to call him incompetent and useless', whereas for extremely small men, 'people mock them and hold

7 See Bondestam, 'An Education', in this volume.
8 Furió Ceriol, *El concejo*, p. 121.

them in low esteem'.[9] This section of *El concejo*, titled 'On the Qualities of the Counsellor Concerning the Body', reveals a striking anxiety regarding anatomic harmony. Yet, this preoccupation with bodily appearance stems from a concern with the beholder's reaction to seeing the body:

> The fourth quality that demonstrates the competence of the counsellor regarding the body is natural proportion, correspondence, and compliance of the limbs, of which there should be neither lack nor excess; either of these defects reveal very bad signs of the soul, and what is more, offend the eye of the beholder.[10]

From this excerpt it seems evident that Furió Ceriol considered that a deviant corporeality implied moral shortcomings. Bodily appearance, according to the Spanish humanist, was evidence of how the soul acted in relation to the body, determining the suitability of the individual for a public position.

Furió Ceriol's ideas – that the human soul acted upon the body and that the physical aspect was an indicator of the quality of the soul – are, in fact, one of two conflicting standpoints regarding the communion of body and soul. In *Theory and History of Ideological Production*, Juan Carlos Rodríguez defines the early modern period as a moment of transition between feudal and bourgeois ideologies, characterized by the continuous dispute for supremacy between the two. This clash of ideologies would lead to the formulation of contending notions, and in particular, that of body and soul. According to Rodríguez, feudal ideology – which he calls *substantialism*, following Gaston Bachelard – was heavily dependent on the hylomorphic doctrine, which claimed that all that existed in the universe was a combination of matter – *materia prima* – and form.[11] This doctrine found one of its strongest advocates in thirteenth-century Dominican theologian Thomas Aquinas, who held that the soul was the substantial form of the human being, and that it informed prime matter so as to compose a single unified substance. Informed by Thomistic hylomorphism, feudal ideology, thus, considered the soul as the informing principle of the body, but never to the extent of becoming visible in it.[12] At the same time, however, by analogy, the human body signified 'worldly existence as a whole, that is, the kingdom of appearances' – which is, clarifies Rodríguez,

9 Ibid., p. 122.
10 Ibid., p. 122.
11 Rodríguez, *Theory and History*, p. 93.
12 Ibid., p. 80.

on the one hand, that which really exists in the here and now and, on the other, 'that from which one must ascend, from one ring to the next, to the perfect forms that give the visible world life'.[13] Rodríguez argues that feudal ideology presupposes the incidence of a spiritual cause on the existence of a similarly organized material order and that, following that logic, 'beauty' signified the perfect influence of the soul on the body. In feudal ideology, the notion of material perfection – or *pulchritudo*, as Rodríguez calls it – designates 'the proportion between the parts, understanding proportion as order and hierarchization or, more precisely, as a whole ordered hierarchically'.[14] Hence, if 'beauty' was considered the harmonic and hierarchical relation or proportion between parts and whole – that is, the perfect influence of the soul on the body – any discordance in this relation, any lack of physical proportion, was 'seen as a ludicrous or dramatic shortcoming'.[15] Without the slightest hesitation, Furió Ceriol's assumptions about applicants with bodily malformations reveal the overwhelming influence of the feudal notion of the relation of cause and effect between body and soul in his thought:

> The integrity of the parts means that a man should not to be born lacking any of them, that means, to be born one-eyed, hunchbacked, lame, without an arm or foot or leg, or marked by the lack or excess of matter, because those who are so born always have ten thousand shortcomings in reason, habits and lifestyle.[16]

When pondering whether he would allow persons with bodily appearances that did not obey the aesthetic canon to form part of the king's council, Furió Ceriol left no room for doubt. His position was not based exclusively on the fact that a deviant body was not able to compel others to pay the respect the position required but, rather, it was based on the idea that physical malformations could betray a poor inclination of the soul and, consequently, were incompatible with the moral rectitude required to legitimize state institutions. According to this logic, a body such as that of Ruíz de Alarcón would be understood as a sign of being informed by a defective soul and that, therefore, would make him inadequate for a position in the state's administrative apparatus.

13 Ibid., pp. 80-81.
14 Ibid., p. 80.
15 Ibid., p. 81.
16 Furió Ceriol, *El concejo*, p. 122.

The body of the playwright

Returning to the report issued by the Council of the Indies regarding Ruiz de Alarcón, the physical imperfection to which the president of the council was referring was in fact a severe malformation of the playwright's spinal column and chest. While scholarship has mostly overlooked Ruiz de Alarcón's precise condition and seems comfortable with merely referring to him as a hunchback, it is possible through careful analysis to determine that the playwright likely suffered from hyperkyphosis, an excessive curvature in the thoracic region of the dorsal spine. This disorder deforms the thoracic vertebrae, which adopt the form of a wedge and cram together, pushing the chest dramatically forward. Visually, the spectacular nature of the arching of his back manifested itself in the form of a protuberant hump. The inclination of his chest was so pronounced that Francisco de Quevedo went so far as to say that Ruiz de Alarcón walked 'breast to calf'. In the *seguidillas* 'A don Juan Ruiz de Alarcón, Corcovado', an anonymous author claimed that the playwright wore 'his belly on his neck'.[17] In effect, the pressure that the posture of Ruiz de Alarcón's dorsal spine was applying on his ribcage squeezed the sides of his breast such that it narrowed and protruded forward in the form of a keel.

It is also known from the writers who assailed the playwright that Ruiz de Alarcón suffered from *genu valgum*, a deformity of the legs. His muscles turned inward, joined at the knees and separated the heels outward. In the satirical *décimas* written as a response to the publication of the *Elogio descriptivo a las fiestas que su Magestad del Rey Filipo IIII hizo por su persona* (1623), Antonio de Mendoza called Ruiz de Alarcón 'the knock-kneed among the poets'. This anomalous curvature of his legs would have caused the unbalancing of his pelvis. The pelvic tilt would have forced his torso to correct his skeletal equilibrium, curving his spine sideways and causing scoliosis. In effect, the curvature of his spinal column would have influenced his stature dramatically. In a report presented in May of 1607 to the Casa de Contratación in Seville, the government agency responsible for the regulation of Spain's trade with its American colonies, Juan de la Torre Ayala appeared as a witness for Ruiz de Alarcón's attempt to gain passage to the Indies. There, he declared that the playwright was of small stature.[18]

17 Reported by Hartzenbusch in the introduction to Ruiz de Alarcón, *Comedias*, p. xxxiv.
18 Rodríguez Marín, *Nuevos datos*, p. 12.

The body as pretext in smearing tactics

The pigeon chest and the hump would establish through their influence the unmistakable signs of Ruiz de Alarcón's identity. These malformations were registered for posterity in the cutting satirical poems with which his literary rivals tried to ridicule him, particularly after the publication of the *Elogio descriptivo*. This poem, which commemorated the festivities celebrated in honour of Prince Charles of England and the Infanta María's nuptials, was commissioned by Don Francisco de Sandoval y Rojas, duke of Cea. The *Elogio* was composed by Ruiz de Alarcón in collaboration with twelve other writers, most of them belonging to the Academy of Madrid. The low stylistic quality of the text, assembled in pieces composed by various authors, presented a perfect opportunity for Ruiz de Alarcón's literary rivals to humiliate him. Not long after the work was published, other works were circulated among the members of the literary academies at court, such as the *Comento contra setenta y tres stancias que don Juan de Alarcón ha escrito* (1623), and a collection of burlesque poems, *Décimas satíricas a un poeta corcovado, que se valió de trabajos ajenos* (1623). Both documents, which underscore the mediocrity of the *Elogio descriptivo*, deride the anatomical defects of the playwright. Indeed, their authors established a direct correlation between the low merit of the poem and Ruiz de Alarcón's physical appearance.

Most of these vexing compositions were *vejámenes*, satirical pieces that were meant to be read out loud in the gatherings of literary academies. The *vejámenes* were originally the closing act of poetic jousts – a competition during which members of the academy would contend to demonstrate their lyric superiority, stirring up rivalries and jealousy – but they were eventually adopted as integral part of any academy session. These jocose compositions consisted in subjecting a peer member to public mockery in order to provoke laughter at his expense. The *vejámenes* were meant to put the finger on the sore spot, touching on sensitive matters such as bodily defects, ethnic origin, social class, moral behaviour or sexual orientation.[19] Some of the participants to whom these compositions were directed would feel so offended that, on occasions, their public reading would degenerate in turbulent scuffles. Even though only a few of them were actually published, the great majority of these compositions were preserved in manuscript form and circulated mainly among participants and attendees. The audience of these pieces consisted not only in the finest writers of the moment, generally followed by an entourage of supporters and aspiring lesser poets,

19 Ferri Coll, 'Burlas y chanzas', I, p. 331.

but also in members of the nobility that would officiate as patrons, as well as other intellectuals such as university scholars. It is natural, thus, that particularly memorable *vejámenes* transcended these groups and were circulated in the court.

Ruiz de Alarcón's presence in such a toxic environment would hardly go unnoticed. The severity of his physical deformity provided his literary rivals with an easy target to pour out their vitriol. Luis de Góngora described him as a tortoise that carried two shells, one on its front and another behind. Luis Vélez de Guevara called him 'dwarf camel,' and Alonso del Castillo y Solórzano said that his humps were on 'front and back.' Francisco de Quevedo, perhaps the author most enraged by Ruiz de Alarcón, revelled in his deformity. In his well-known satirical poem 'Corcovilla' he used the image of shoulder blades made of a barber's shaving bowl in order to describe Ruiz de Alarcón's torso. In short, a barrage of all sorts of insults fell on the playwright. His enemies issued all kinds of epithets to him: 'frog', 'ape', 'half-dwarf' and 'embryo', among dozens of other names.

The public abuse of the figure of Ruiz de Alarcón included, to a lesser or greater degree, the most illustrious writers of the age: Lope de Vega, Luis Vélez de Guevara, Francisco de Quevedo and Luis de Góngora. While we do not know if or to what extent these attacks would have affected Ruiz de Alarcón, by April 1625 he did not appear among those aggravated by Anastasio Pantaleón de Rivera's 'Vejamen de Sirene', at the 1625 gathering of the Academia de Medrano, a detail that suggests that he had already stopped attending those meetings.[20] By that time, the position request that Ruiz de Alarcón had made to the Council of the Indies was already under revision.

The scene of resistance

Juan Ruiz de Alarcón was no stranger to this type of abuse. Soon upon his return to the Iberian Peninsula, in 1613, the playwright had began to experience antagonism as he became a conspicuous presence in the royal court setting. Ruiz de Alarcón's persistent efforts to build support from courtly patrons and, ultimately, to obtain a position in the state administration, stirred jealousy in his rivals. In 1617, Luis Sánchez's printing workshop published *El pasajero*, by Cristóbal Suárez de Figueroa. Suárez de Figueroa, who displayed a profound aversion to Ruiz de Alarcón, was a former judge in Teramo, Naples, who had returned to the Iberian Peninsula thirteen years

20 King, *Juan Ruiz de Alarcón*, p. 185.

before and was also struggling to pursue an administrative position. Suárez de Figueroa's purpose in *El pasajero*, a novel written as a dialogue between four travellers, was to denounce the moral relaxation of Spanish society and to propose a reform of customs and habits. Following a discussion on the appointment of *regidores* – the highest-ranking officials in a municipal government – in which one character outlines the preferable bodily features that an applicant should present, Suárez de Figueroa makes an unmistakable reference to Ruiz de Alarcón, justifying the playwright's debarment from any public position:

> If the midget, although well-formed and able, should find rejection in that which he desires – if he is to represent authority with his person – there are many more reasons for the ape in the shape of a man, the imprudent hunchback, the grotesquely deformed one forgotten by God, to find rejection when pursuing some public office.[21]

Perhaps significantly, this early recorded instance of verbal abuse against Ruiz de Alarcón coincides with the playwright's first steps as writer of dramatic works. It is of course difficult to determine whether the cutting commentaries dumped on him in *El pasajero* – which probably were neither the first, not the only ones – had a major influence on the composition of *Las paredes oyen*. Whatever drove Ruiz de Alarcón to write this play, it is undeniable that *Las paredes oyen* was ultimately conceived as a plea for resisting and challenging the bodily representational regime in vogue in seventeenth-century Spanish society – and the Hapsburg administrative system, for that matter.

The earliest known account of the staging of *Las paredes oyen* – and of any other play written by Ruiz de Alarcón – dates from 3 February 1618, when two of the playwright's dramas, *Las paredes oyen* and *Los favores del mundo*, were being staged in the church of Our Lady of Victory's convent in Madrid.[22] *Las paredes oyen* must have been composed, thus, before that date, that is, at some point during the four years after Ruiz de Alarcón's return to the Iberian Peninsula.

At the heart of the action in *Las paredes oyen* is a love triangle formed by Don Juan de Mendoza and Don Mendo de Guzmán, who are rivals for the love of Doña Ana de Contreras, a young widow. Both male characters represent the antitheses of one another: while Don Juan is a middle-aged

21 Suárez de Figueroa, *El pasajero*, p. 425.
22 Cotarelo y Mori, 'Las comedias'.

man, poor and whose physical appearance is hinted to be deviant, Don Mendo embodies the ideal of the seducer, 'handsome, rich, and young' ('*bello, rico y mancebo*') (v. 70). Each character, however, is the opposite of what he looks like. Whereas Don Juan's actions reflect his noble character, Don Mendo articulates his relationship with the rest of the characters through lies, a means that he exploits in an almost pathological way, even resorting to violence in order to reach his goals. Similar to the Spanish aphorism 'lies have short legs,' Doña Ana will disabuse herself of Don Mendo as she goes about unravelling his lies. Don Juan de Mendoza's moral qualities will finally make Doña Ana fall in love with him, the most unlikely love interest.

The character of Don Juan de Mendoza awakened the fascination of those critics who have approached *Las paredes oyen*. 'Poor and ugly / and *malformed*' ('*pobre y feo / y de mal talle*'; the italics are mine) (vv. 11-12), though of noble origin, Don Juan de Mendoza seems to be an avatar of the author himself, with which he shares not only the name – the playwright signed as Juan Ruiz de Alarcón y Mendoza – but also misfortune. The enigmatic '*mal talle*' with which the character of Don Juan defines himself is, likewise, the reason for which the gentleman is rejected by the woman he loves.

Doña Ana's first words in *Las paredes oyen* are triggered by the uncontrollable aversion she experiences at the sight of Don Juan. Upon entering the room where her suitor awaits her, the widow cannot contain her disgust and, in an aside, blurts out to her maid, 'oh, Celia! What an ugly face / and bad shape Don Juan has!' ('*¡ay, Celia, y qué mala cara / y mal talle de don Juan!*') (vv. 195-196). Doña Ana confesses as much to Celia a little later: 'How can I love / a man whose face and shape / annoy me just on sight?' ('*¿Cómo puedo yo querer / hombre cuya cara y talle / me enfada solo en miralle?*') (vv. 942-944). The aside with which Doña Ana makes her entrance in the play puts the audience into a privileged position: the spectator, a mute witness to the seductive ploys employed by the hapless lover, is always aware that this is a lost battle and cannot help but feel sorry for him. Don Juan's point of departure invariably places him at a disadvantage, since he constantly has to overcome the first irrational and involuntary reaction to the sight of his ugliness. The unfolding of events will, however, soften Doña Ana's position.

In *Las paredes oyen*, the rejection that Don Juan's bodily appearance provokes in Doña Ana begins to weaken thanks to a conversation that the young widow overhears accidentally. Scene 13, Act I – according to the stage directions – opens with the actresses playing the part of Doña Ana and her maid, Celia, standing behind a window, and three other actors representing the roles of Don Juan, Don Mendo and the duke of Urbino down in the street. It is dark outside and the two women are behind a lattice screen. Neither can Doña Ana and Celia clearly see the group of men, nor can the three men see the women from the outside. Doña Ana, who is preparing for a trip to Alcalá de Henares with Celia, notices a group of men gathered in front of her balcony, and she overhears that they are talking about her. She recognizes the voices of her beloved Don Mendo, accompanied by Don Juan and a third gentleman, the duke of Urbino. Concealed behind the latticework window of the balcony, she listens, stunned, to the debate that her two suitors are having over her beauty. Although the opinions of both men regarding the beauty of the widow coincide, Don Mendo, who is wary of awakening the duke's interest in the widow, feigns scorn towards her and paints a regrettable portrait of Doña Ana. Stupefied, she cannot believe the words of her beloved. Her surprise grows upon realizing that the only member of the group that defends her is Don Juan. The contorted man does not skimp on praises, exalting the beauty of Doña Ana before the duke who, to Don Mendo's despair, expresses a desire to meet such a sublime beauty. The duke's determination obliges Don Mendo to exaggerate his speech, uttering more ignominies, which Doña Ana listens to indignantly.

The obscurity of the night prevents Doña Ana from clearly seeing the group of men, while the lattice screen keeps her and her maid out of sight of the group of men. The lattice screen, a decorative device, the function of which is to provide privacy while allowing the person inside to observe the outside, serves as a physical boundary between Doña Ana's room – the domestic space, reserved for women – and the street – the social space, the domain of men. While it is not an optic device, in a sense, the lattice screen behaves like a visual filter, allowing the observer to see or preventing the outsider from seeing through it. Because of the absence of light, Doña Ana cannot see the group of men, but she is able to identify each one of them by their voices. The lattice screen functions in this scene as a device that renders the visible invisible and the invisible visible. In the darkness of night, filtered through the lattice screen, the appearance of the men's bodies dissolves. What Doña Ana witnesses is the pure essence of the men – their naked souls, free from the constraints of their bodies. By eliminating Don Mendo's handsomeness, the lattice screen reveals his mean spirit. In the same way, once the malformed body of Don Juan is removed from the field of view, the beauty of his soul presents itself before Doña Ana in all its splendor.

It is clear that Ruiz de Alarcón's understanding of the soul and its relationship to the body is at odds with that of Furió Ceriol. As it is palpable in the construction of the characters of Don Juan and Don Mendo, the incidence of a spiritual cause – that is, their 'souls' – on matter – their bodies – does not presuppose an exact equivalence in terms of a hierarchical and harmonious proportion between parts and whole, nor does it necessarily mean that the body is a mirror image of the soul, and vice versa. If anything, for Ruiz de Alarcón, the body operates as an envelope that conceals the soul and prevents it from being noticeable, and the soul can only be apprehended through its expressive force. According to Juan Carlos Rodríguez, this formulation of the influx of the soul into the body corresponds with bourgeois ideology – or *animism*, as he calls it.[23] Rodríguez considers that the former coincides with the social construction of the figure of the poet, that is, in his own words, that of 'the artist of genius' who 'is capable of capturing and exposing [...] the interior form which beautiful souls possess'.[24] As a result, the task of the poet would be that of the 'extraction of the idea hidden in the matter'.[25] Therefore, the body, argues Rodríguez, is an essential requirement for the *animist* dialectic. As Rodríguez puts it, 'the extraction of the idea hidden in matter implies not the suppression of matter but rather its spiritualization', that is, rendering the body 'a transparent expression of the interior soul'.[26] What is at stake, argues Rodríguez, is the expressive liberation of the poet's sensibility – that is, his soul. Thus, following that logic, liberating the soul consists in rendering the body transparent.[27] Scene 13, Act I of *Las paredes oyen* puts a twist on this notion. Here the expressive force of the characters' souls is only made visible, paradoxically, by means of opacity. Instead of rendering Don Juan and Don Mendo's bodies transparent, Ruiz de Alarcón buries them in obscurity, so that physical appearance does not divert attention from the observation of the soul.

The character of Don Juan de Mendoza can be considered of particular significance to scholars interested in the intersection of early modern literature and disability studies. In effect, few characters of the period submerge both readers and spectators alike in the social experience of being marginalized on account of possessing a deviant bodily appearance. More importantly, to my knowledge, Don Juan represents the first case – and perhaps the only one – of an early modern disabled character conceived by an author with a disability, that is, created from the embodied experience of being in a disabling world. Don Juan's disability, however, does not manifest

23 Rodríguez, *Theory and History*, p. 74.
24 Ibid., p. 74.
25 Ibid., p. 74.
26 Ibid., p. 78.
27 Ibid., p. 78.

itself in the play as a physical or intellectual limitation. Instead, Don Juan possesses an extraordinary command of the spoken word, and a lyricism far superior to that of his rival Don Mendo. In fact, the reader only knows Don Juan's physical deformity thanks to the scant allusions made to his physical aspect over the course of the play. What would be perfectly obvious for the playgoers, who would see before them a Don Juan moving awkwardly across the stage, would go completely unnoticed for the reader if it was not for the scant textual references to his outward aspect.

As a matter of fact, it seems difficult for the reader to see this paragon of virtue as a loathsome creature. The reader of the play experiences the same epiphany as Doña Ana, both being removed from the visual contemplation of the malformed body of the protagonist. Both Doña Ana and the viewer are transported to another plane of perception in which the essence of the characters is received in a more vibrant form, without the interference of aesthetic taste. Ruiz de Alarcón must have been completely conscious of the disparate effect that reading the *comedia* would produce, compared to seeing it performed upon a stage. This could be one of the main reasons for which he hastened to publish *Las paredes oyen* in the first volume of his plays (1628). The truth that *Las paredes oyen* tried to show was perhaps achieved more effectively through its reading than through its staging. As the text suggests, Ruiz de Alarcón intends to go beyond merely illustrating the process of ignoring bodily appearance: his purpose was to activate in the reader the capacity to perceive what lies beyond the perceptible. *Las paredes oyen* speaks to a truth hidden behind the appearance of matter. So that this truth may be contemplated unencumbered by bodily assumptions, the appearance that covers it must be ignored. In short, one must get rid of the body.

Conclusion

Ruiz de Alarcón's erasure of the body crashed head-on with the attitude of the Hapsburg administrative apparatus. As demonstrated by the 1625 report that evaluated Ruiz de Alarcón's aptitude for a position in the Royal Audiences of the American colonies, the Council of the Indies was not concerned with the Mexican playwright's capabilities as a lawyer. What really made the colonial administration uneasy was the way in which his admission might affect the institution's public image.

During a span of twelve years, until Phillip IV's ascent to the throne in 1621, the Council of the Indies systematically rejected Ruiz de Alarcón's continuous applications. Despite enjoying royal protection in 1625, the playwright still could not persuade the council to grant him the position requested. Like Suárez de Figueroa, Juan de Villela, president of the Council of the Indies, considered that Ruiz de Alarcón's physical appearance could lead to complications when it came to imposing the necessary respect to the authority of the office. Villela preferred to grant Alarcón an ecclesiastic job in the Indies or a position as *relator*, a judicial clerk at the council. The *relator* position had the advantage of working in private, free from public scrutiny. *Relatores* practiced their profession in the entrails of the bureaucratic apparatus. Their main role was to summarize documentation to be presented before judges and governors so that they did not have to face litigants.[28] In the opinion of Villela, this was the ideal job for Ruiz de Alarcón. Phillip IV must have agreed, since, in response to the report, he signed his own name and stated 'alright, and when you have the chance, you, the president, will grant him a position as judicial clerk'.[29]

On 17 June 1626, Phillip IV would finally name Ruiz de Alarcón supernumerary judicial clerk, a post which he would ultimately acquire and occupy until his death in 1639. Consequently, Juan Ruiz de Alarcón's efforts to obtain an administrative post in accordance with his level of legal education had concluded. While it would be legitimate to claim that Ruiz de Alarcón never obtained the appeals court position he strived for, his appointment as *relator* at the Council of the Indies was far from being a saddening defeat. Playwrights who were more notorious and better connected than him, such as Lope de Vega – who was unsuccessful in securing the position of Royal Chronicler for himself – or Miguel de Cervantes – who had been declined several bookkeeping positions in the American colonies – had failed to do so. In exchange for the post, Ruiz de Alarcón consented that his body, malformed and poorly treated by age and illness, be hidden from public scrutiny. He might have had the satisfaction of knowing that, in reality, it had been the beauty of his verses that had won him his post. Thanks to his plays, he enjoyed the admiration of Ramiro Núñez de Guzmán, son-in-law of the prime minister, the count-duke of Olivares, who would become his most steadfast protector. Like his character, Don Juan, the playwright's soul had triumphed over his body. Once he had achieved the post of *relator*, Ruiz de Alarcón would never again write plays.

28 Bermúdez Aznar, 'El oficio de Relator', p. 430.
29 Fernández-Guerra y Orbe, *Don Juan Ruiz de Alarcón*, p. 523.

Works Cited

Bermúdez Aznar, Agustín, 'El oficio de Relator del Consejo de Indias (siglos XVI-XVII)', in *Derecho, instituciones y procesos históricos, tomo I: XIV Congreso del Instituto Internacional de Historia del Derechi Indiano*, ed. José de la Puente Brunke and Jorge Armando Guevara Gil (Lima: Pontificia Universidad Católica del Perú, 2008), pp. 429-456.

Cotarelo y Mori, Emilio, 'Documentos. La madre de Lope de Vega. Los padres del autor dramático don Juan Ruiz de Alarcón', *Boletín de la Real Academia Española* 2 (1915), pp. 525-526.

Cotarelo y Mori, Emilio, 'Las comedias en los conventos de Madrid en el siglo XVII', *Revista de la Biblioteca, Archivo y Museo* 8 (1925), pp. 461-470.

Fernández-Guerra y Orbe, Luis, *Don Juan Ruiz de Alarcón y Mendoza* (Madrid, 1871).

Ferri Coll, José María, 'Burlas y chanzas en las academias literarias del Siglo de Oro: Los Nocturnos de Valencia', in *Actas del XIII Congreso de la Asociación Internacional de Hispanistas, Madrid 6-11 de julio de 1998*, ed. Florencio Sevilla Arroyo and Carlos Alvar Ezquerra, 4 vols (Madrid: Castalia, 2000), vol. 1, pp. 327-335.

Furió Ceriol, Fadrique, *El concejo, y consejeros del príncipe* (1559), in *Obra completa I: El concejo y consejeros del príncipe; Bononia*, ed. Henry Méchoulan and Jordi Pérez Durà (Valencia: CNRS Universitat de Valencia, 1996), pp. 83-135.

Kagan, Richard L., *Students and Society in Early Modern Spain* (Baltimore: Johns Hopkins University Press, 1974).

King, Willard F., *Juan Ruiz de Alarcón, letrado y dramaturgo* (México: El Colegio de México, 1989).

King, Willard F., 'La ascendencia paterna de Juan Ruiz de Alarcón y Mendoza', *Nueva Revista de Filología Hispánica* 19, no. 1 (1970), pp. 49-86.

La Barrera y Leirado, Cayetano Alberto de, *Nueva biografía de Lope de Vega*, vol. 1 of *Obras completas de Lope de Vega* (Madrid: Real Academia Española, 1890).

Maravall, José Antonio, *Estado moderno y mentalidad social* (*Siglos XV a XVII*), 2 vols (Madrid: Editorial Revista de Occidente, 1972).

Maravall, José Antonio, 'Los "hombres de saber" o letrados y la formación de su conciencia estamental', *Estudios de historia del pensamiento español*, 3 vols (Madrid: Ediciones Cultura Hispánica, 1973-1975), vol. 2, pp. 355-389.

Rangel, Nicolás, 'Noticias biográficas del dramaturgo mexicano D. Juan Ruiz de Alarcón y Mendoza. Nuevos datos y rectificaciones', *Boletín de la Biblioteca Nacional de México* 11, no. 1 (1915), pp. 1-24.

Rodríguez, Juan Carlos, *Theory and History of Ideological Production* (Newark: University of Delaware Press, 2002).

Rodríguez Marín, Francisco, *Nuevos datos para la biografía del insigne dramaturgo D. Juan Ruiz de Alarcón* (Madrid, 1912).

Ruiz de Alarcón, Juan, *Comedias de Juan Ruiz Alarcón y Mendoza*, ed. Juan Eugenio Hartzenbusch (Madrid, 1852).
Ruiz de Alarcón, Juan, *Obras completas*, 3 vols, ed. Agustín Millares Cano (México: Fondo de Cultura Económica, 1996).
Suárez de Figueroa, Cristóbal, *El pasajero*, ed. María Isabel López Bascuñana, 2 vols (Barcelona: Promociones y Publicaciones Universitarias, 1988).
Vega, Lope de, *Comedias escogidas de Frey Lope Félix de Vega Carpio*, ed. Juan Eugenio Hartzenbusch (Madrid, 1860).
Vincens Vives, Jaume, *Coyuntura económica y reformismo burgués* (Barcelona: Editorial Ariel, 1968).

About the Author

Pablo García Piñar is a lecturer at Cornell University and he specializes in early modern Spanish literature and disability studies. He is currently working on a book-length study on disability in transatlantic Golden Age Spain, tentatively entitled *Unfit for Office: Normativity and the Embodiment of State Authority in Early Modern Spanish Literature*.

4. 'The Most Deformed Woman in France': Marguerite de Valois's Monstrous Sexuality in the *Divorce satyrique*

Cécile Tresfels

Abstract
The anonymous satirical *Divorce satyrique* (1660) stages the fake confession of Henri IV, king of France, who justifies his divorce from Marguerite de Valois by her monstrous sexuality, describing her as 'the most deformed woman in France'. This chapter explores how sexuality and monstrosity are linked to representations of feminine power within the context of general satire against the Valois family during the French Wars of Religion. Additionally, it shows how this violent pamphlet is symptomatic of a transitional period in which the definition of monstrosity evolves from physical to internal abjection. This cultural transition allows the writer to bring the sexual shaming of a woman to a new misogynistic level that essentializes the concept of female depravity.

Keywords: early modern women, slut-shaming, monster studies, sexuality studies, Henri III, Catherine de Medici

The *Divorce satyrique*, an anonymous satirical piece written around 1607 and published in 1660,[1] stages the fake confession of Henri IV, king of France, who justifies his divorce from his ex-wife Marguerite de Valois by the monstrosity of her sexuality: '*un siecle moins vicieux s'esmerveillera que le notre ait*

1 First published in *Recueil de diverses pièces servans à l'histoire de Henri III* [...] (Cologne: Pierre du Marteau, 1660). I will use the version published in D'Aubigné, *Oeuvres complètes*. This version contains the additions of 1663 that mention the existence of two illegitimate children that will not be studied in this essay. The translations are mine and the text will be abbreviated as DS in the notes.

Bondestam, M. (ed.), *Exceptional Bodies in Early Modern Culture: Concepts of Monstrosity before the Advent of the Normal*. Taylor & Francis Group, 2020
DOI 10.5117/9789463721745_CH04

produit un monstre au lieu d'une femme'[2] (a less perverted century than ours will marvel at the fact that ours produced a monster in lieu of a woman). Marguerite was not the only member of the Valois family whose sexuality had been described as monstrous by her detractors during the French Wars of Religion. Her brother, Henri III, was attacked for his alleged homosexual relationships with his 'mignons' in numerous satirical pieces gathered in Pierre de L'Estoile's *Registre-journal*.[3] Her mother, Catherine de Medici, was depicted in *Le Réveille-matin des Français* as 'a sexually corrupting "*putain*" who was determined to control the king by introducing him to sexual debauchery, especially sodomy'.[4] More generally, sexual attacks were a common political weapon in the conflict between protestants and Catholics.[5] Marguerite herself had previously been the target of a few of them,[6] but never with such violence. Unlike Henri, Marguerite was a woman and unlike her mother, she was childless. The *Divorce satyrique* used the specificity of this status to build a monstrous representation that combined an excessive and deviant sexuality with the lack of legitimate children.

The power of this satirical piece, in addition to its violence, lies in the fact that it adopts a biographical approach, depicting the evolution of Marguerite's sexual practices temporally and geographically, a technique that had previously been used against Catherine de Medici in the *Discours merveilleux* (1576).[7] It follows the queen from her marriage to Henri de Navarre in Paris, to Agen, to Carlat, to her years of exile in Usson and finally back to Paris where she returned after her divorce, and when the *Divorce satyrique* was written. The text overuses referentiality to actual people, places and anecdotal details to reinforce its claim for veracity. According to Éliane Viennot, only seven of the endless amount of lovers listed can be considered as having been loved by or having loved Marguerite.[8] However, the writer seems to have an excellent knowledge of Marguerite's life from the years 1574 to 1575, 1579 to 1586 and 1606 to 1607, which serves the goal of the satire to blur the boundary between fact and fiction.[9] This aim was

2 DS, p. 666.

3 Ferguson, *Queer (Re)Readings*; Long, *High Anxiety*.

4 Crawford, *Sexual Culture*, p. 11. See also Chang and Kong, *Portraits*; McIlvenna, *Scandal and Reputation*.

5 Viennot, *La France*, pp. 652-659.

6 Viennot, *Marguerite de Valois*, pp. 313-320.

7 Chang and Kong, *Portraits*.

8 Guise, La Mole, Bussy, Champvallon, Aubiac, Dat and Bajaumont. See Viennot, 'Agrippa d'Aubigné', p. 98.

9 Ibid., p. 99.

accomplished to the extent that this piece has been adopted as a historical biographical source by writers and historians, which led to the construction, over the centuries, of the myth of the libidinous and mischievous *Reine Margot*.[10] The text mentions for example that Marguerite had incestuous relationship with her brothers, and that she buried the head of her beheaded lover La Mole, two inventions that will fuel the legend over the centuries.[11] The monstrosity of this piece thus also resides in the history of its misogynist reception, which has deformed Marguerite de Valois into a caricatural figure, while contributing to the delegitimization of her status as a writer.

This is ironic considering that the main target of the *Divorce satyrique* seems to have been Henri IV, presented as a coward, an impotent and lacking agency in the different political stages of the Wars of Religion. The double satire of the *Divorce satyrique* relies indeed on the traditional misogynistic trope of the excessive, unruly, disorderly woman and of the weak man, unable to control her.[12] Typical arguments against women such as the ones found in witchcraft treatises or in the *Querelle des femmes* are used to present Marguerite as an all too typical woman: carnal, inconsistent and prone to follow her passions.[13] However, it paradoxically presents her as exceptional, exceeding all previous models. What constitutes her monstrosity is the fact that her sexuality goes against nature (incest), against her rank (lovers from low extraction), against religion (extramarital intercourse and sodomy, defined as nongenerative sexual practices) but especially against established expectations on the conduct of and respectability for women. In the *Divorce satyrique*, Marguerite's body is presented as transgressing all boundaries: it is extensible, penetrable, unstoppable, it oozes and it consumes, and thus it profoundly disturbs. The violence of the attack against Marguerite's sexuality is illustrative of the anxieties that such transgressions raise: Marguerite becomes a Protean character who calls into question gender distinction, class distinction, the divide between human and animal, and upper and lower bodily strata, which is seen as destabilizing and threatening. This chapter will explore how ordinary misogyny and depictions of the exceptional work together in the *Divorce satyrique* to create a monstrous representation of Marguerite that had long-lasting consequences on the reception of her historical character.

10 Viennot, *Marguerite de Valois*; Sealy, *The Myth*.

11 Viennot, *Marguerite de Valois*, pp. 320-325.

12 Davis, 'Women on Top'.

13 Kramer, *Malleus Maleficarum*. For the *Querelle des femmes*, see Dubois-Nayt, Dufournaud and Paupert, *Revisiter*.

What has been at the centre of literary critics' investigation is the attempt to establish the authorship of the *Divorce satyrique*. Several suggestions have been made: Jean Choisnin, Scipion Dupleix, Palma Cayet, Charles de Valois or Agrippa d'Aubigné.[14] Going hand in hand with this question of authorship, what has also preoccupied the critics is the 'literariness' of the text. According to several of them, it is because it contains passages deemed quite brilliant that its attribution to a great canonical author such as D'Aubigné is made possible. Another aspect of the research on the *Divorce satyrique* has been to study its reception and to explore the role it played in the construction of the myth of the *Reine Margot*.[15] However, no study to date has approached this text through the lens of monstrosity. This chapter thus wishes to underline how sexuality and monstrosity are linked to representations of feminine power within the context of general satire against the Valois family. Additionally, it will show how the *Divorce satyrique* is symptomatic of a transitional period in which the definition of monstrosity evolves from external to internal abjection. This cultural transition of the monstrous allows the writer to bring the sexual shaming of a woman to a new misogynistic level that essentializes the concept of female depravity.

Naming and characterizing the monstrous whore

Marguerite de Valois is first mentioned via a periphrasis: '*celle dont l'infamy a longuement obscurcy ma reputation*'[16] (the one whose infamy has long obscured my reputation). By not naming her directly, the narrator already distances himself from her and makes vileness the main element of her character. Her name only appears a few paragraphs later but in the words of Charles IX, that he allegedly pronounced before her wedding with Henri IV: '*il protestoit soubs mille serments, qu'il ne donnoit pas sa Margot seulement pour femme au Roy de Navarre, mais à tous les Heretiques de son Royaume*'[17] (he swore a thousand times that he did not only give his Margot as wife to the king of Navarre but also to all the heretics of his kingdom). The narrator

14 Viennot, 'Agrippa d'Aubigné'; Dubois, 'Le *Divorce satyrique*'. D'Aubigné is seen as the most probable author and the text has been added to D'Aubigné's *Oeuvres* in the edition that we are using for this contribution, with the reluctance of the editor but following the suggestion of several critics. See D'Aubigné, *Oeuvres*, p. 655.

15 Viennot, *Marguerite de Valois*; Sealy, *The Myth*.

16 DS, p. 656.

17 Ibid., p. 657.

considers this sentence as proleptically foreshadowing his wife's fate as national whore. By using the familiar nickname 'Margot' preceded by the possessive '*sa*' (her) in the words of her brother Charles IX the narrator also refers, from the very beginning of the pamphlet, to the accusation of incest between Marguerite and her brothers.[18] She is then referred to throughout the text via ironic antiphrases that are supposed to underline the discrepancy between what she is supposed to be: '*une Princesse, fille, soeur et femme de Roy*'[19] (a princess, daughter, sister and wife of a king) and what she actually is: '*un monstre au lieu d'une femme*'[20] (a monster instead of a woman). The narrator thus calls her successively '*la pucelle*'[21] (the virgin); '*ma preude femme*'[22] (my prude wife); '*ma chaste femme*'[23] (my chaste wife); '*ceste preude femme*'[24] (this prude woman); '*ceste vertueuse princesse*'[25] (this virtuous princess), revealing the norms against which her sexuality is assessed, in order to underline what she is not.

In the middle of the text, her identity is reduced to the part of her body that the entire satire focuses on, also representing this part as diseased and contagious through a grotesque and disgusting image: '*c'est le plus puant & le plus infect trou de tous ceux qui pissent*'[26] (it is the most infectious and reeking of pissing holes). At the end of the text, describing the way Marguerite dresses when she goes to church to receive communion, the narrator uses the following terms:

> osant impudemment depuis plusieurs années trois fois la semaine faire sa Pasque dans une bouche aussi fardée que le cœur, la face plastrée & couverte de rouge, avec une grande gorge descouverte qui ressembloit mieux & plus proprement à un cul, que non pas à un sein[27]
> (daring impudently for several years and three times a week to receive communion in a mouth as painted as her heart, her face plastered and covered in red, with a great bosom so uncovered that it resembled rather an ass than breasts)

18 The expression '*sa Margot*' is also from the *Réveille*, as well as the mention of the incest with one of her brothers. See Viennot, *Marguerite de Valois*, p. 314.
19 DS, p. 665.
20 Ibid., p. 666.
21 Ibid., p. 659.
22 Ibid.
23 Ibid., p. 660.
24 Ibid., p. 669.
25 Ibid.
26 Ibid., p. 667.
27 Ibid., p. 676.

Running the metaphor of the 'hole' and pairing it with an upside-down effect (her buttocks are where her breasts should be), the narrator transforms Marguerite's entire body into a single function, the one of being penetrated.

This characterization is complemented by a series of powerful, blasphemous and grotesque comparisons to objects and animals that paint the portrait of the aforementioned deformed body. She is first compared to mercury, a metal that becomes liquid at room temperature, and that has the ability to wet other metals: '*aussi mouvante que le Mercure elle bransloit pour le moindre object qui l'approchoit*'[28] (as moving as mercury, she swayed for every object that approached her). Her sexual approachability and availability then takes the form of the offertory box at church:

> [I]l n'estoit point fils de bon lieu, ni gentil compagnon, qui n'avoit une fois en sa vie eesté serviteur de la Royne de Navarre, qui ne refusoit personne, acceptant ainsi que le tronc publicq les offrandes de tous venans.[29]
> ([T]here wasn't any son of a good place, nor a kind companion, that had not been once in his life servitor of the queen of Navarre, who never refused anyone, accepting, like the offertory box at church, the offerings of all.)

Marguerite's body is thus characterized as shapeshifting, porous to its surroundings and penetrable ad infinitum. And these intrinsic qualities define her promiscuity, a relationship that is at the basis of the sexual shaming rhetoric operated by the narrator. Animal metaphors are also used to underline her bestiality and the baseness of her sexual practices:

> mais estant mal aisé que le poisson ne revienne à l'hameçon, & le corbeau à la charogne, ce haut-de-chausse à trois culs se laisse derechef emporter à la lubricité & débordée sensualité[30]
> (but knowing that the fish always comes back to the hook, and the crow to the carcass, these three-ass breeches let themselves be carried away again by lubricity and overflowing sensuality)

28 Ibid., p. 659. Up to the seventeenth century '*bransler*' meant primarily to move inconsistently and could also mean to hesitate. Bransler: 'To brandle; totter; shake, swing; shog, wag, reele, stagger; waue, wauer; nod often, stirre apace, moue vncertainely, or inconstantly, from side to side; also, to tremble, or quake. Cotgrave, *A Dictionarie of the French and English Tongues*. Even if a sexual meaning existed in the sixteenth century it started to refer to sexual intercourse in the seventeenth century and more generally to masturbation in the nineteenth century. For an analysis of the term in Montaigne's *Essays*, see Calhoun, 'Montaigne's *Branloire*'.

29 DS, pp. 661-662.

30 Ibid., p. 665.

The narrator also blasphemously compares her starving belly to the one of the biblical whale and himself to Jonas[31] and her sexual appetite is compared to the one of a bloodhound.[32] These three animal metaphors underline the constant drive that animates a body that is never full. The effects of this particular imagery are numerous and work on different registers. If the farcical nature of breeches with the capacity for three asses can lead to laughter, the combination of allusions to a decomposing and deformed body, as well as to the threats of a hunting dog and a starving whale convey disgust but also fear. What makes her behaviour so fearful is the fact that it is presented as relentless and totalizing.

The word '*putain*' (whore) is mentioned at the very end of the pamphlet as part of a song written by someone on the door of the 'Hostel de l'Evesque de Sens' where she spent the night upon her return to Paris: '*Comme Roine elle devoit ester / Dedans la Royale maison: / Mais comme putain c'est raison, / Qu'elle soit au logis d'un prestre*'[33] (As queen she should have been in the royal House; but as whore it makes sense that she should stay at a priest's). The insult is developed by the narrator directly in the following paragraph in which he underlines '*son inclination au putanisme*'[34] (her inclination to whoring) after having named her '*la plus difforme femme de France*'[35] (the most deformed woman in France). Marguerite's sexual monstrosity is thus first established through a series of denominations that, explicitly or by antiphrastic contrast, underline the immorality of her sexual behaviour as well its grotesque physicality.

Monstrous behaviour: Excessive and unnatural

But why is Marguerite so monstrous according to the narrator? Let us first consider definitions of monstrosity in the sixteenth and seventeenth centuries in order to understand what the concept might mean for the anonymous writer of the satire and its readers. According to Wes Williams, monstrosity is first related to an extraordinary physical appearance.[36] The aforementioned comparisons, presenting her as shapeshifting and taking metaphorically the form of objects and animals, are one way to convey her monstrosity.

31 Ibid., p. 666.
32 Ibid., p. 668.
33 Ibid., p. 679.
34 Ibid., p. 681.
35 Ibid.
36 Williams, *Monsters*.

Marguerite's peeling skin is another physical element in the text that contributes to the portrait of a monstrous body. As underlined by Lorraine Daston and Katharine Park, medical particularities in the Renaissance fascinated physicians and the readers of their accounts.[37] Towards the end of the text,[38] the narrator describes the medical strategies she had to use during intercourse because of the skin disease she suffered from: erysipelas, also referred to as St. Anthony's Fire because of the intensity of the rash that it causes. It appears on the body as red, swollen, hot and shiny patches and was thought up until the seventeenth century to be caused by high blood temperature and an excess of choleric humour. The depiction of a sick body performing sexual activities contributes to the monstrous physical characterization of Marguerite.

But throughout the *Divorce satyrique*, Marguerite's deformed and sick body is presented much more as the consequence, the sign, of a monstrous behaviour, rather than monstrous in itself.[39] External appearance is indeed not what constitutes Marguerite's monstrosity per se. Rather, it is the use that she makes of her body that is considered unnatural, and it is this repetitive unnatural use of her body throughout time that gradually has consequences on her external appearance. Monsters and marvels are defined in the following terms by Ambroise Paré, famous surgeon of the time, in his treatise and catalogue *Of Monsters and Prodigies*:

> Monsters are things that appear outside the course of Nature (and are usually signs of some forthcoming misfortune), such as a child who is born with one arm, another who will have two heads, and additional members over and above the ordinary. Marvels are things which happen that are completely against Nature as when a woman will give birth to a serpent, or to a dog.[40]

Monstrosity, in Paré's sense, is evaluated quantitatively ('*outre Nature*') whereas marvels' criteria are qualitative ('*contre Nature*'). Monsters are defined

37 Daston and Park, *Wonders of the Order of Nature*, p. 145.

38 DS, p. 684.

39 See the depiction of Richard III by Thomas More, in which the deformed body is related to deviant morality, in Cohen, 'Monster Culture', p. 9; Garber, *Shakespeare's Ghost Writers*, p. 30. Pablo García Piñar also develops this relationship between a deformed body and deviant morality: 'From this excerpt it seems evident that Furió Ceriol considered that a deviant corporeality implied moral shortcomings. Bodily appearance, according to the Spanish humanist, was evidence of how the soul acted in relation to the body, determining the suitability of the individual for a public position.' García Piñar, 'The Optics of Bodily Deviance', in this volume.

40 Paré, *On Monsters*, p. 3.

by a supernumerary excess, and marvels by an antinomy. The depiction of Marguerite's sexuality in the *Divorce satyrique* fits in both categories. The first thing that constitutes her monstrosity is quantitative. The large number of her sexual encounters is expressed under the form of lists or totalizing expressions. Her lovers are enumerated at the beginning of the text and the narrator apologizes about some possible chronological confusion: '*car le nombre m'excusera si je fauls à les bien ranger*'[41] (they are so numerous that you will have to forgive me if I do not list them in the right order). Several passages suggest that she had sexual relationships with every single man in the kingdom of France and her exile in Usson is then described as a 20-year-long orgy:

> [E]lle se resoud de n'obeïr qu'à ses volontez, & d'establir dans ce Roc l'Empire de ses délices, où clause de trois enceintes & tous les grands portaux murez, Dieu sçait & toute la France les beaux jeux qui en vingt-ans se sont jouëz & mis en usage.[42]
> ([S]he decided to only obey her own will and to establish in this castle the empire of her delights, where, surrounded by three walls and solid gates God and the entire country know the wonderful games that, in 20 years, were played and invented.)

The assumption that the entire country of France is already aware of what allegedly happened behind Usson's gates functions as a rhetorical manipulative move that allows the author to create a form of complicity with its readers while making up fictitious witnesses.

The second element that makes her even more monstrous is the socially unacceptable qualitative aspect of these sexual encounters: the diversity of her lovers' social status. The discrepancy between the height of her rank and the lowness of her countless lovers constitutes, according to the narrator, the most shocking aspect of her sexual practices. The *Divorce satyrique* thus traces the itinerary of a social demotion through sexuality, from the Gascogne Cadets to the mule-drivers and coppersmiths of Auvergne. As we progress geographically, the social status of her lovers gets lower and lower. Her exile in Usson, where she is described as having sex with her domestics and secretaries, constitutes the nadir of this downgrading:

> [C]'est bien loin de ce que sa bonne fortune luy promettoit, l'ayant fait naistre d'un des plus grands & Magnanimes Roys de la terre, de la voir

41 DS, p. 660.
42 Ibid., pp. 673-674.

> aujourd'huy valeter de la sorte, & tellement reduitte du trot au pas, que de Royne elle soit venuë Duchesse, & de legitime Espouse du Roy de France, amante passionnée de ses valetz.[43]
> ([I]t is far from what her good fortune promised her, being born from the grandest and most generous kings of the earth, and now serving others, and so reduced from trot to walk, that from queen she became duchess and from legitimate wife of the king of France, passionate lover of her servants.)

Her monstrosity is thus both quantitatively and qualitatively defined, bringing together Paré's definitions of monsters and marvels.

This qualitative social aspect is complicated by a focus on gender transgression: Marguerite's lovers are sometimes portrayed as challenging masculine conventions, which is seen as contributing to the overall monstrosity of her sexual practices. They either blend with her by their femininity, or they are feminized by her in order to better suit her desire.[44] For example, the narrator describes the transformation that Canillac undergoes when he becomes the queen's lover, becoming much more effeminate and polished than he used to be.[45] The same Canillac is mocked by the narrator for being used by Marguerite for political purposes, before being dismissed. But one lover in particular embodies an ambiguous masculinity that is seen as perverse: Pominy. Described as appearance-shifting and always hiding furtively, he was the son of a coppersmith and made his way to the queen through singing, before becoming one of her secretaries. He is described as a key step in the degradation of Marguerite's sexual practices:

> [C]'est pour luy que les folies se sont si fort augmentées, qu'on en pourroie fournir des justes volumes: c'est de luy qu'elle dit qu'il change de corps, de voix, de visage, & de poil, comme il luy semble: & qu'il entre à huis clos où il luy plaist.[46]
> ([I]t is for him that her extravagances grew so much that one could write entire volumes about them: she says she is the one who changes bodies, voices or hair as he pleases, who enters in enclosed spaces as he wishes.)

43 Ibid., p. 676.

44 On gender and the redefinition of masculinity in the early modern period, see Long, *High Anxiety*; Reeser, *Moderating Masculinity*. On gender, sexuality and the Valois family, see Laguardia, 'Henri III'.

45 DS, p. 672.

46 Ibid., p. 674.

Shapeshifting and ubiquitous, this fluid character is supposed to illustrate the degeneration of Marguerite's sexuality.

Last but not least her monstrosity lies in the misuse of her reproductive ability.[47] Marguerite never gave Henri a child, which played a big part in their separation. What the *Divorce satyrique* conveys is that Marguerite was so sexually active that she 'wasted' her body's reproductive capacity. In a paragraph devoted to fecundity and impotence, the couple's reproductive power is assessed by the narrator. Henri, who had been said to have smelly feet and to be impotent, brags about his numerous illegitimate children, and assures the reader he does not know why sexual encounters with Marguerite did not lead to the conception of a child. However, in the next sentence, he confesses that Marguerite unwillingly had sex with him but willingly did so with a 'thousand' others, thus presenting this overuse of her body as the cause of their mutual infertility:

> [M]ais je n'ay sceu onques deviner la cause de nostre compagnie sterile & infructueuse, ni pû l'attribuer aux raisons communes, bien que je sçache qu'à regret elle a souvent consenty à la force de mes desirs pour se donner volontairement en proye à mille.[48]
> ([B]ut I have never been able to guess the cause of our sterile and fruitless company, nor could attribute it to the usual reasons, although I know that she often consented regretfully to the strength of my desire in order to willingly offer herself to a thousand.)

The text thus implicitly establishes the fact that a woman's body gets used up the more she uses it. Marguerite, by unwillingly having sex with her husband but willingly with others, is portrayed as sinful because her reproductive function was not put to proper use.[49]

So not only is Marguerite's body described as shapeshifting and physically repulsive but her appearance and behaviour are presented as destabilizing everyone around her as well as the social, religious and political order. She

47 Read, *Birthing Bodies*; McTavish, *Childbirth*. The importance of the distinction between a bodily activity and the purpose of this activity for the regulation of exceptional movements is also underlined by Maria Kavvadia: 'It was not the body activity per se that was criticized; rather, it was the purpose and the circumstances under which a body activity was practiced that defined it as appropriate or not.' Kavvadia, 'The *Moresca* Dance in Counter-Reformation Rome', in this volume.

48 DS, p. 669.

49 See Chang and Kong, *Portraits*: 'the queen's ability to produce an heir secured her place and her own political capital', p. 3.

calls into question categories of gender, social status, but also inheritance and reproduction.[50] In doing so, we can say that she is described as resolutely disorienting, and thus queer, in the sense developed by Sara Ahmed in *Queer Phenomenology*. Marguerite complicates indeed 'the relationship between inheritance (the lines that we are given as our point of arrival into familial and social space) and reproduction (the demand that we return the gift of the line by extending that line)'.[51] A childless and divorced queen in the sixteenth century defies the expectations associated with this status, and it is not surprising that the *Divorce satyrique* was written at the time where Marguerite, back in Paris, and renamed 'Queen Marguerite', was thriving as the leader of an artistic and intellectual court.[52] By making this exceptional status monstrous, the text actually reveals the gendered social and political anxieties that are raised when faced with 'lines [that] might be marks of the refusal to reproduce: the lines of rebellion and resistance that gather over time to create new impressions on the skin surface or on the skin of the social'.[53]

External and internal monstrosity

If quantity and quality are used to depict Marguerite's sexuality, the tension between exteriority and interiority is the ultimate tool used by the narrator to establish her behaviour as morally monstrous and to make Marguerite's monstrosity inherent to her being. In a single sentence, the narrator synthesizes the main causes of this monstrosity that we previously analysed (range, diversity and nature). He lists the number of sexual encounters: '*infinies amours*' (infinite loves), the nature of her desire: '*conceuës par un sale désir, guidé par l'effronterie, entretenuë par la volupté*' (conceived by an immoral desire guided by impudence and fuelled by delight), and the diversity of its manifestations: '*ainsi que ces deshonnestes plaisirs, dont la diversité vous estonne, & le vice augmente mon deshonneur*' (as well as these dishonest pleasures, whose diversity shocks you and whose vice increases my dishonour).[54] The qualifying

50 'This refusal to participate in the classificatory "order of things" is true of monsters generally: they are disturbing hybrids whose externally incoherent bodies resist attempts to include them in any systematic structuration.' Cohen, 'Monster Culture', p. 6.

51 Ahmed, *Queer Phenomenology*, p. 17.

52 See Viennot, *Marguerite de Valois*, pp. 263-304.

53 Ahmed, *Queer Phenomenology*, p. 18.

54 DS, pp. 670-671.

adjectives in the expressions '*sale désir*' and '*deshonnestes plaisirs*' show that Marguerite's sexuality is considered morally monstrous. Throughout the text, the narrator makes a point of underlining that this monstrosity comes from within and that this extraordinary sexuality is driven by an internal desire. Her deformed body is a consequence and manifestation of this internal monstrosity, reflecting materially the depravity of her soul. And this internal monstrosity is related to pleasure, sought, found and renewed. The narrator of the *Divorce satyrique* uses several expressions belonging to the lexical field of interiority as related to morality: '*inclination à la volupté*'[55] (inclination to pleasure); '*son naturel inconstant qui se lasse de tout*'[56] (her inconstant nature that gets tired of everything), and goes even as far as saying that he could devote another piece to '*les monstruositez de son esprit*'[57] (the monstrosities of her soul). This transfer of the notion of monstrosity from the outside to the inside throughout the sixteenth and seventeenth century is underlined by Williams: 'By the late seventeenth century the term "*monstrueux*" is more likely to denote hidden intentions, unspoken desires. [...] Put most schematically, monsters move off the maps and into the home, move from being literally out there, other in some external sense, to being metaphorically in here, interior, constitutive of the self.'[58] The *Divorce satyrique* exemplifies this shift, as Marguerite's monstrous sexuality is presented as coming from an internal desire, constitutive of her being.

But the text goes even further and depicts Marguerite as gradually internalizing the fact that she is perceived as a monster, and even perceives herself as such. As a consequence, she tries to hide this monstrosity, which makes her slowly lose her mind, and, from dominating, she becomes dominated. This switch is made explicit in the lexical transition between 'affections' and 'foiblesses' towards the end of the text: '*Tant & si diversifies sont et ont esté jusques ici ses affections, ou plustost ses foiblesses* (*car ainsi faut-il baptizer ses jalousies et dernieres fureurs amoureuses*)'[59] (So diverse were her affectations, or rather her weaknesses, since one has to name as such her jealousies and latest love furies). From then on, Marguerite is presented as a victim of her dishonest passions and the accusations of the narrator shift to a different realm. The first one is the accusation of noncoincidence

55 Ibid., p. 662.
56 Ibid., p. 666.
57 Ibid., p. 682.
58 Williams, *Monsters*, p. 1.
59 DS, p. 676.

between the inside and the outside, which is a key feature of monstrosity according to Michael Uebel:

> Monsters, as discursive demarcations of unthought, are to be treated not exclusively as the others of the defining group or self, but also as boundary phenomena, anomalous hybrids that constantly make and unmake the boundaries separating interiority from exteriority.[60]

Henri underlines several times the discrepancy between her pious appearance and her lack of faith. And, at the end of the text, this discrepancy becomes Marguerite's principal and totalizing characteristic: '*En somme tout son fait n'est qu'apparence & ostentation, sans aucune estincele de devotion ni de pieté: Je la connois de longue main*'[61] (In sum, her whole being is only appearance and ostentation, without a sparkle of devotion or piety: I have known her long enough to know). This accusation of duplicity have precedents in the attacks against Henri III, who was accused of having a secret life behind closed doors and behaving differently in public.[62] But it is also to be found in the *Discours merveilleux*, the most virulent pamphlet against Marguerite's mother Catherine de Medici, that portrays her 'maliciousness,' a direct consequence of her Florentine origins.[63]

This duplicity is depicted as having consequences on Marguerite's mental health towards the end of the satire:

> [N]e pouvant quelquefois parmi la pitié que j'en ay m'empescher de rire des extravagantes jalousies, & fortes passions qu'on raconte de ses amours, qui la transportent plus souvent à mespriser ce qu'elle voit, & à croire ce qui n'est point.[64]
> ([A]nd sometimes I cannot help myself, in spite of the pity that I feel, to laugh at her extravagant jealousies and at the strong passions that I hear of her loves that transport her very often to despise what she sees and to believe what is not.)

The verb '*transporter*' points to an uneasiness of the soul and an increasing lack of agency caused by the strength of her passions, leading to paranoia and

60 Uebel, 'Unthinking the Monster', p. 266.
61 DS, p. 682.
62 Ferguson, *Queer (Re)Readings*, pp. 317-318.
63 Chang and Kong, *Portraits*, p. 47.
64 DS, p. 677.

hallucinations. Furetière's dictionary (1690) defines 'transport' as a medical term related to the displacement of humours, but also as a moral term, indicating the agitation of the soul by the violence of the passions. Going back to the figure of Pominy, the narrator depicts Marguerite as completely obsessed with him, carrying around her neck in Usson a blue purse containing his portrait, that he ordered her to never remove nor open. After having been described as a seductive manipulator, the queen is now portrayed as a pitiful victim, lacking agency. After having depicted her sexual encounters externally, the narrator scrutinizes Marguerite internally and progressively develops the idea that Marguerite herself becomes conscious of her own monstrosity. He depicts, for example, a process of internalized shame that makes Marguerite blush when she hears the words '*honneur*' and '*vertu*'.[65] In Usson, during her exile that is presented as 'voluntary,' she is depicted as constantly afraid and suspicious of her own self, because of the conscience she had of her immorality:

> Il n'est point de juge meilleur que la conscience, elle nous esveille & nous poind ordinairement en la partie la plus dolente: aussi cette Dame [...] s'est renduë subjecte à ne pouvoir plus tolerer qu'on tousse, rie, ou parle bas en sa presence, tant le soupçon & le mefy d'elle-mesme luy fait apprehender le discours de ses actions.[66]
> (There is no better judge than our conscience, she awakens us and presses usually on our most doleful part: hence this lady [...] made herself unable to tolerate that one coughs or laugh or speaks in a low voice in her presence, since the suspicion and distrust that she has for herself makes her apprehensive of what will be said of her actions.)

By making Marguerite ashamed of her own monstrosity, the narrator presents her as the own victim of her immoral sexual behaviour. The *Divorce satyrique* is thus symptomatic of a transitional period in which the definition of monstrosity evolves: Marguerite is shamed not only for acting like a whore but for being one to the core.

Conclusion

The most monstrous aspect of this text, however, lies in its gendered and enduring reception. The purpose of this double satire was, as we mentioned

65 Ibid.
66 Ibid.

in the introduction, twofold: debasing the husband, the king, via the monstrosity of the wife's sexuality. The author of the text aimed primarily to impair the reputation of the once-protestant king. Throughout this defence, Henri is indeed presented as a coward who admits that he knew about his wife's infidelities but chose to accept them since they were serving his own interests: '*sa beauté m'attiroit force Gentil hommes, et son bon naturel les y retenoit*'[67] (her beauty allowed me to attract several gentlemen and her good nature made them stay). He even presents himself as an accomplice at some point, reading with Marguerite the letters that Pibrac sent her.[68] More serious accusations are also to be found in the text: Henri is depicted as a traitor who gave up his protestant faith and not only forgave his enemies, but ended up trusting them:

> J'ay pardonné à plus d'ennemis que vengé d'injures, [...] n'ayant pas absous seulement les perturbateurs de l'Etat de leur crimes, mais aussi remis mon particulier intérest à ceux qui, téméraírement, ont osé attaquer mon nom.[69]
> (I have forgiven more enemies than I have avenged offenses [...] having not only absolved the perturbators of the state of their crimes, but also put my own interest in the hands of those who, audaciously, dared to attack my name.)

More generally the depiction of the king's wife's monstrous sexuality allows the author to attack the king's masculinity and nobility, whose rivals were from a much lower social status and who was the only one that Marguerite slept unwillingly with.

However, the rhetorical strategy of the pamphlet ironically presents the narrator, Henri IV, as aiming for the opposite goal: the restoration of his reputation and the justification of his divorce. Referring to this text as a '*Manifeste*', he hopes for his words to last for centuries to come.[70] His wish came true indeed since it is for Marguerite de Valois that this satire had the most durable and impactful consequences. The *Divorce satyrique* has been a work of reference for novelists such as Stendhal in 1830 with *The Red and the Black* (in which the heroine Mathilde de La Mole worships Marguerite for burying the head of her lover) or Dumas in *La Reine Margot*

67 Ibid., p. 661.
68 Ibid., p. 662.
69 Ibid., p. 656.
70 Ibid., p. 675.

(1845), movie directors such as Patrice Chéreau (who portrays incestuous relationships between Marguerite and her brothers in *La Reine Margot*,[71] which received the Prix du Jury at the Cannes Film Festival in 1994), but also, and more problematically, for many biographers, historians and literary critics. A similar confusion between the biographical and the legendary have fuelled the problematic reception of other figures of feminine power, such as Catherine de Medici, previously mentioned, but also Marie Antoinette.[72] As Susan Broomhall states, '[w]omen in positions of power were not only unsettling to contemporaries, but continue to provoke strong feelings in those who have crafted narratives of the past'.[73] It is this problematic reception, in addition to the historical and cultural context in which these pamphlets were produced, that we need to keep investigating in order to understand the ongoing association of exceptional women with monstrosity.

Works Cited

Ahmed, Sara, *Queer Phenomenology: Orientations, Objects, Others* (Durham: Duke University Press, 2007).

Aristotle, *Generation of Animals*, trans. Arthur Leslie Peck (Cambridge, MA: Harvard University Press, 1963).

Broomhall, Susan, 'Feelings for Powerful Women', *Histories of Emotion: From Medieval Europe to Contemporary Australia* [blog], 29 July 2016. https://historiesofemotion.com/2016/07/29/feelings-for-powerful-women/ (accessed 22 July 2020).

Calhoun, Alison, 'Montaigne's *Branloire*: Passage, Impact, Vibrant Matter', *Montaigne Studies* 30 (2018), pp. 29-39.

Castle, Terry, 'Marie Antoinette Obsession', *Representations* 38 (1992), pp. 1-38.

Chang, Leah L., and Katherine Kong, *Portraits of the Queen Mother: Polemics, Panegyrics, Letters* (Toronto: Centre for Reformation and Renaissance Studies/Iter, 2014).

Cohen, Jeffrey Jerome, 'Monster Culture: (Seven Theses)', in *Monster Theory: Reading Culture,* ed. Jeffrey Jerome Cohen (Minnesota: University of Minnesota Press, 1996), pp. 3-25.

Cotgrave, Randle, *A Dictionarie of the French and English Tongues* (London, 1611).

71 Viennot, 'À propos'.

72 Price, 'Vies privées'; Castle, 'Marie Antoinette Obsession'; Crawford, 'Constructing Evil'; Hunt, 'The Many Bodies'.

73 Broomhall, 'Feelings for Powerful Women'.

Crawford, Katherine, 'Constructing Evil Foreign Queens,' *Journal of Medieval and Early Modern Studies* 37, no. 2 (2007), pp. 393-418.

Crawford, Katherine, *The Sexual Culture of the French Renaissance* (Cambridge: Cambridge University Press, 2010).

Daston, Lorraine, and Katharine Park, *Wonders of the Order of Nature, 1150-1750* (New York: Zone Books, 1998).

D'Aubigné, Agrippa, *Oeuvres complètes de Théodore Agrippa d'Aubigné: publiée pour la première fois d'après les manuscrits originaux accompagnées des notices biographiques, littéraires & bibliographique, de variantes, d'un commentaire, d'une table des noms propres & d'un glossaire* (Paris: A. Lemerre, 1873).

Davis, Natalie Zemon, 'Women on Top', in *Society and Culture in Early Modern France: Eight Essays* (Stanford: Stanford University Press, 1975), pp. 124-151.

Dubois, Claude-Gilbert, 'Le *Divorce satyrique* de la Reyne Marguerite', in *Marguerite de France, reine de Navarre, et son temps: actes du colloque d'Agen, 12-13 octobre 1991*, ed. Madeleine Lazard et al. (Agen: Le Centre Matteo Bandello d'Agen, 1994). pp. 99-106.

Dubois-Nayt, Armel, Nicole Dufournaud and Anne Paupert, eds, *Revisiter la Querelle des femmes. Discours sur l'égalité/inégalité des femmes et des hommes, de 1400 à 1600* (Saint-Etienne: Publications de l'Université de Saint-Etienne, 2013).

Ferguson, Gary, *Queer (Re)Readings in the French Renaissance: Homosexuality, Gender, Culture* (Aldershot: Ashgate, 2008).

Garber, Marjorie, *Shakespeare's Ghost Writers: Literature as Uncanny Causality* (New York: Routledge, Chapman & Hall, 1988).

Huet, Marie Hélène, *Monstrous Imagination* (Cambridge, MA: Harvard University Press, 1993).

Hunt, Lynn, 'The Many Bodies of Marie Antoinette: Political Pornography and the Problem of the Feminine in the French Revolution', in *Eroticism and the Body Politic*, ed. Lynn Hunt (Baltimore: Johns Hopkins University Press, 1991), pp. 108-130.

Laguardia, David, 'Henri III et la propagande de l'obscène', *Réforme, Humanisme, Renaissance* 68 (2009), pp. 41-52.

Long, Kathleen P., *High Anxiety: Masculinity in Crisis in Early Modern France* (Kirksville: Truman State University Press, 2002).

McIlvenna, Una, *Scandal and Reputation at the Court of Catherine de Medici* (London: Routledge, 2016).

McTavish, Lianne, *Childbirth and the Display of Authority in Early Modern France* (Aldershot: Ashgate, 2005).

Niccoli, Ottavia, *Prophecy and People in Renaissance Italy* (Princeton: Princeton University Press, 1990).

Paré, Ambroise, *On Monsters and Marvels* (Chicago: University of Chicago Press, 1982).

Price, Leah, 'Vies privées et scandaleuses: Marie Antoinette and the Public Eye', *The Eighteenth Century* 33, no 2 (1992), pp. 176-192.
Read, Kirk D., *Birthing Bodies in Early Modern France: Stories of Gender and Reproduction* (Farnham: Ashgate, 2011).
Reeser, Todd W., *Moderating Masculinity in Early Modern Culture* (Chapel Hill: U.N.C. Department of Romance Languages, 2006).
Sealy, Robert J., *The Myth of the Reine Margot: Towards the Elimination of a Legend* (New York: Peter Lang, 1994).
Spinks, Jennifer, *Monstrous Births and Visual Culture in Sixteenth-Century Germany* (London: Routledge, 2016).
Uebel, Michael, 'Unthinking the Monster: Twelfth-Century Responses to Saracen Alterity', in *Monster Theory: Reading Culture*, ed. Jeffrey Jerome Cohen (Minneapolis: University of Minnesota Press, 1996).
Viennot, Éliane, 'Agrippa d'Aubigné, Marguerite de Valois et le *Divorce satyrique*', *Albineana* 7 (1996), pp. 87-111.
Viennot, Éliane, 'À propos du film de Patrice Chéreau: *La Reine Margot* ou la modernité inculte', May 1994. https://web.archive.org/web/20131211192859/http://elianeviennot.fr/Articles/Viennot-MgV-Chereau.pdf (accessed 22 July 2020).
Viennot, Éliane, *La France, les femmes et le pouvoir I: L'Invention de la loi salique (Ve-XVIe siècle)* (Paris: Perrin, 2008).
Viennot, Éliane, *Marguerite de Valois: 'La reine Margot'* (Paris: Perrin, 2005).
Williams, Wes, *Monsters and Their Meanings in Early Modern Culture: Mighty Magic* (Oxford: Oxford University Press, 2011).

About the Author

Cécile Tresfels is Assistant Professor of French at Williams College. Her research focuses on the interplay of cognition and emotion in the early modern period and on the intersection of gender, sexuality and politics during the French Wars of Religion. She also develops inclusive pedagogies for second-language acquisition.

5. Curious, Useful and Important: Bayle's 'Hermaphrodites' as Figures of Theological Inquiry

Parker Cotton

Abstract

This essay examines Pierre Bayle's use of the hermaphrodite figure in his *Dictionnaire.* Bayle repeatedly connects the hermaphrodite to mythic tales and language, rather than engaging 'real' accounts of intersexed persons. Bayle's hermaphrodite functions as an entry point into theological discussions of sin and leads his readers across articles considering a hermaphroditic first man ('Adam') and the potential for humans unmarred by sin ('Sadeur'). The hermaphrodite is employed as a sceptical figure to aid in raising questions and becomes part of a larger Baylean challenge to a dogmatic and rigid theology of the age. Bayle's hermaphrodite articles and the questions of human nature he raises within them demonstrate how discussions of exceptional bodies contribute to ongoing theological debates in the early modern period.

Keywords: human nature, mythic, prelapsarian, scepticism, scripture, subversion

In the *avertissement* of the August 1684 issue of his *Nouvelles de la république des lettres,* Pierre Bayle (1647-1706) defended his choice to avoid descriptions of 'monsters', amongst other scientific subjects, saying: 'it is not that these things are not very curious, very useful or very important' but rather these subjects are covered by similar works. Bayle had a specialized project in mind and largely kept the *Nouvelles de la république des lettres* covering philosophical and theological works despite the popularity of some 'curious' subjects. Born in France, Bayle moved to Rotterdam amidst increasing

Bondestam, M. (ed.), *Exceptional Bodies in Early Modern Culture: Concepts of Monstrosity before the Advent of the Normal.* Taylor & Francis Group, 2020
DOI 10.5117/9789463721745_CH05

pressure upon Protestants from the French authorities and remained there in exile after the Revocation of the Edict of Nantes (1685). Yet even in the relatively tolerant Dutch Republic his writings stirred up trouble. Bayle's most famous work, his *Dictionnaire historique et critique* (1697) is notorious for his articles dealing with the problem of evil, bringing Bayle under fire from the Walloon Church for suggesting there is no rational solution for how God and evil can coexist.[1] Consisting of massive volumes of alphabetized articles, the *Dictionnaire* contained much of its inciting material in the sprawling footnotes, named 'remarks' by Bayle. Here one finds the philosopher offering comments, often of sensational aspects of stories, on the more factual main articles and connecting themes across articles by a vast series of cross-references. By the time the *Dictionnaire* appears Bayle not only covers popular, curious subjects but actively seeks out controversial and thought-provoking figures of theological inquiry.

This essay began as an investigation into Bayle's use of monsters in the *Dictionnaire*, trying to determine how his embrace of popular subject matter may have changed from the earlier *Nouvelles de la république des lettres*. Provocative comments are commonplace throughout the *Dictionnaire*, yet often appear in a 'throwaway' manner. Bayle will insert a risqué reference in a single remark of a much larger article and have no larger connections to such comments. However, the hermaphrodite content does not follow this pattern.[2] Rather, we see Bayle link whole articles to remarks which detail hermaphrodites. Although these remarks may initially seem to be naughty comments to capture readers' attention, I believe they share some larger thematic concerns which Bayle wants to explore.[3] I will situate Bayle alongside the stream of thought which employed the hermaphrodite as a subversive figure. More particularly and uniquely, I argue that this subversiveness was attached to theological ideas through Bayle's featuring of the hermaphroditic figure in doctrinally charged articles of the *Dictionnaire*.

I will first offer some background on how hermaphrodites were viewed in the early modern period, and the changing historiography of marvels. Next, the layout of the *Dictionnaire* and how it may have functioned will be explained before walking through the articles with more prominent

1 See Labrousse, *Bayle*, for a succinct English language biography.

2 I retain the period use of 'hermaphrodite' to refer to intersexed persons. This term's connection to the Hermaphroditus and Salmacis myth helps to emphasize my interest in Bayle's subversive use of the intersex figure, and Bayle's lack of reference to 'real' bodies.

3 One of, if not the most, popular works of the eighteenth century, Bayle's *Dictionnaire* owes much of its success to the controversies and obscenities it promoted. See Lennon and Hickson, 'Pierre Bayle'.

hermaphrodite references. Following this, I shall discuss the role of the hermaphrodite as a sceptical figure in the early modern period. The idea of the hermaphroditic body drew attention to, and related concepts of, subversion and scepticism through it's 'disordering' of nature. I demonstrate how Bayle picks up on this usage and employs the hermaphroditic body to open questions of theological importance. The exceptional body challenges the established orthodoxy.[4]

Early modern hermaphrodites

In order to situate some of the challenges surrounding Bayle's mythic usage of the hermaphrodite some brief context on the use of hermaphroditic and monster language in the early modern period is required. The traditional tale offers a developmental picture of rational thought coming to maturity and abandoning the identifying of wonders and monstrosities with the supernatural.[5] This narrative has been complicated by recognition of the persistence of wonder in various modes.[6] The term 'monster' may be used for a wide variety of wonders regardless of whether the speaker seeks to capture natural or supernatural elements. Hermaphrodites can operate as both natural figure and supernatural sign and any distinction we may want to make becomes blurred as monsters are considered in the early modern period. Ruth Gilbert demonstrates with reference to the title of Ambrose Paré's 1573 text *On Monsters and Marvels*[7] that although Paré thought monsters were aberrations of nature whereas marvels were something wholly unnatural, the term 'monster' can both designate horror or the awe-filled marvellous. This notion of awe in considering positive perspectives on monsters maintains the disruptive factor common to horror that we may not associate with our common understanding of marvel. Monsters in this positive light were signs to grab attention.[8]

4 See Bondestam, 'An Education', in this volume, for how tangible and unique specimens can serve a similar role in challenging reflections on normalcy. See also Moore, 'Monsters and the Maternal Imagination', in this volume, for how the human body is juxtaposed (and manipulated) with the monstrous, disrupting assumptive interpretations.

5 Park and Daston, 'Unnatural Conceptions'.

6 Daston and Park, *Wonders*. Daston and Park amend their earlier developmental view with this more complicated account of normalization.

7 Gilbert, *Early Modern Hermaphrodites*, p. 25.

8 Ibid., pp. 21-24. See also Graille, *Les Hermaphrodites*, pp. 34-43, for the history of these views in the early modern period.

Thomas Laqueur has argued that the early modern period saw many people conceive of the human race as only possessing one sex, more perfectly expressed as male. Most people could be easily determined as male or female.[9] This perspective helpfully explains the contradictory positive and negative views of hermaphrodites throughout this period. The hermaphrodite (allegedly) has a choice within this one sex system to display male or female. Philip Almond notes that despite a one sex understanding, one that we may assume makes the hermaphrodite more natural, 'the hermaphrodite *was* a monster or prodigy, a sign of the wrath of God, or at least a point of departure for moral observations on human sin'.[10] Regardless of how we conceptualize early modern constructions of sex, the hermaphrodite remains a problematic figure for classification. If the hermaphrodite cannot be fully comprehended within natural categories, assigning a divine purpose to the body is an easy jump to make.[11] And yet, if this purpose is found (or thought) not miraculous, the view of the hermaphroditic figure seems biased towards the negative as an observation on sin and what has happened to the human body in its fallen state.

Three medical treatises emerged in close succession detailing the intersexed body. Jacques Duval's *Treatise on Hermaphrodites* (1612), Jean Riolan's *Discourse on Hermaphrodites* (1614) and Gaspard Bauhin's *On the Nature of Births of Hermaphrodites and Monsters* (1614). In each the authors focused on figuring out *what* was happening in these bodies, particularly around questions of generative potential.[12] The hermaphrodite undergoes increased cataloguing in an attempt to order it as an understandable, if not natural, phenomenon. The concerns of the hermaphroditic body as disrupting society remained, but were approached from a different angle, the 'scientific'.[13] I will return to this societal disruption of the hermaphrodite once we have learned how Bayle uses the hermaphroditic figure for his own disrupting purposes. For now, we note that Bayle, aware of both popular and medical discourse of the preceding century, does not engage this medical literature on hermaphrodites. This was a conscious decision to use the hermaphrodite as a mythic figure.

9 Laqueur, *Making Sex*, p. 124; Almond, *Adam and Eve*, p. 8.

10 Ibid.

11 Cf. Daston and Park, *Wonders*, pp. 122, 221-226; Long, *Hermaphrodites*, pp. 49-75; DeVun, 'The Jesus Hermaphrodite'.

12 See Daston and Park, 'The Hermaphrodite', p. 420.

13 Cf. Long, 'From Monstrosity', pp. 35-41. Long demonstrates that early modern thought also has a tradition of viewing difference as normative.

Reading practice

How Bayle's *Dictionnaire* is meant to be read is a puzzling question. One would never read straight through article after article arranged alphabetically. Yet the dense system of cross-references running throughout the body, comments and notes of articles indicates more than a massive collection of stand-alone articles. Bayle has designed a complex system of information where one can spend hours bouncing between linked articles. Determining the 'final' word on a theme or set of articles is nearly, perhaps intentionally, impossible. Still, a logic can be found between cross-references, and a rough understanding of what themes connect articles can be realized. Small, seemingly insignificant articles connect with some of the most infamous in the *Dictionnaire* to emphasize an elusive Baylean point. Elsewhere, massive 'webs' of interconnected figures can be traced popping in and out of dense discussions. The articles are not stand-alone entries, and what the references are trying to indicate is crucial for interpreting Bayle's work.[14] Further, the footnotes or 'remarks' which Bayle attaches to each article are truly spin-offs, often larger than the article itself. Bayle grants himself the freedom to engage any topic which is even marginally related to the larger article and expand on it at large within these remarks. Here we often find the most interesting and provocative comments in all of Bayle's writings. Even small remarks attached to large articles may contain the briefest of mentions of controversy for no other reason than to engage the controversial.

Mara Van der Lugt's recent work on the interlacing of articles in the *Dictionnaire* has been immensely helpful in visualizing this project, particularly this conception of the articles as 'webs'. Van der Lugt offers a variety of case studies within Bayle's *Dictionnaire* for illustrating the importance of reckoning with webs of articles, rather than taking them as stand-alone entries for interpretation.[15] These webs allow the hermaphroditic cross-references to function together as leading the reader along and into linked themes of inquiry. Returning to our 'hermaphrodite' articles, I want to suggest an entry point to the hermaphroditic web – the 'Adam' article. Bayle generally spent more time constructing the earlier letters of the alphabet, speeding up his writing as the daunting size of the *Dictionnaire* became apparent.[16] Relatively large, the 'Adam' article is indicated as a central point in the web less by size alone than by the number of articles referenced within

14 Van der Lugt, *Bayle*, p. 32.

15 Ibid., pp. 45-46.

16 Ibid., p. 18. See also Van Lieshout, *The Making.*

it. How does one start this journey into Bayle's hermaphrodite articles? By following that great motivator of human behaviour, sin. For the reader interested in the ongoing debates on the nature of original sin, it is hard to think of a more obvious article than 'Adam' to turn to in their copy of the *Dictionnaire*.

Walking through this web will see us move through three main articles tied together: 'Adam', 'Sadeur' and 'Salmacis', with additional cross-references to both 'Eve' and 'Bourignon'. Given the entry point of 'Adam', we find readers following the hermaphroditic breadcrumbs throughout Bayle's writings are walking the path of an open discussion of sin. Sin thus sets a backdrop for the questions Bayle's recounting of hermaphrodite myths will provoke. If this assumption holds, the Baylean hermaphrodite is a figure closely tied to and employed for theological discourse.

'In the beginning' – the 'Adam' article

Bayle reflects on the description of the first man, Adam, provided by the mystic Antoinette Bourignon (1616-1680).[17] Bourignon believed that Adam was created with 'the Principles of both Sexes in himself, and the Power of producing his Likeness, without the help of a Woman.'[18] Some noteworthy points of engagement emerge from this description. First, Bourignon believed that sexual union for the sake of procreation emerged only after the Fall of man, for before this, Adam had the power of procreation himself.[19]

For Bayle, this is 'a gross mistake of the words of Scripture to imagine any such thing'.[20] That is, from the words 'Male and Female he created them' in Gen 1:27, we are not to infer that Adam was created both male and female as Bourignon and others in the kabbalistic tradition would hold. It is a misinterpretation of Scripture to assume that this is a single, hermaphroditic being in view here. What Bayle does not say, however, is that it is an error on behalf of God, or that a hermaphroditic Adam (or person in general) is a divine mistake. His argument against this view is textual. Bayle emphasizes this criticism of Bourignon's interpretation in remark F, restating his view as, 'We need only be able to read the Scripture, to confute

17 For more detail on the 'Adam' article, see Bost, 'Bible et fables'.
18 Art. 'Adam', Rem. G.
19 See DeVun, 'Heavenly Hermaphrodites'. DeVun traces the importance of the hermaphroditic Adam for theological questioning regarding creation and the resurrection of bodies.
20 Art. 'Adam'.

all those chimerical Notions.'[21] It is not appropriate to construct a creation narrative of an intersexed first person when other, more natural, readings of the same text will suffice.[22]

Elsewhere in Bayle's corpus we see him arguing the opposite hermeneutical principle, that is, that the 'plain' or natural reading of Scripture is problematic and must be rejected. This is the position he takes with regard to Luke 14:23 ('Compel them to come in') in the *Philosophical Commentary*. Briefly, this verse had been used, building off Augustine, to justify persecution in order to prompt conversion. Bayle opens the commentary by stating his guiding principle: 'That all literal Construction, which carries an Obligation of committing Iniquity, is false.'[23] In the *Philosophical Commentary*, interpretations which lead us to sin should be submitted to the tribunal of the natural light of reason and reinterpreted, possibly moving away from a literal or common-sense reading, in order to avoid readings that result in wrongdoing. Presumably, Bayle's argument from Scripture in the 'Adam' article works in the opposite direction. The plain reading of the verse, which is, that male and female were created as we know them, separate and distinct, is acceptable as is. It does not lead to iniquity and thus does not need to be reinterpreted. This verse passes the tribunal of reason in a literal reading.

Sadeur

The article 'Sadeur' details the travel account published anonymously by Gabriel de Foigny titled *La Terre Australe connue* (1676) and relates the voyages of one Jacques Sadeur who, while claiming to be a hermaphrodite himself, alleges that the inhabitants of *Terra Australis* also possess both sexes. These Australians treat the single-sexed as monsters, even 'stifling them at birth.' The hermaphrodite Australians are thus positioned as in opposition to the European world and its normalcy of being single sexed. Now, Bayle approaches this story with his typical scepticism and takes care to inform his reader that it is being recorded and mentioned only to

21 Art. 'Adam', Rem. F. The language of 'chimerical' is a common phrase for Bayle and other writers of the time. It is unlikely to bear significance to the discussion of monsters.

22 Patrick Graille thinks that it is Bayle 'perverting' the interpretation of Scripture in this passage. While Bayle restricts the range of interpretation, viewing the literal sense as appropriate, Graille does not provide reasons for delineating proper interpretation from perversion. See Graille, *Les Hermaphrodites*, p. 39.

23 Bayle, *A Philosophical Commentary*, p. 66.

give supplement to what was earlier stated in the 'Adam' article and the views of Antoinette Bourignon, that is, to contribute to the discussion of hermaphrodites.

What is not clearly spelled out is why this discussion should be continued if this travel account of Australia and Sadeur is fictional if not fraudulent. It seems as though Bayle wishes to continue discussing the nature of 'monsters' and how from the perspective of Sadeur's Australians, the 'monsters' are actually culturally abnormal Europeans. The perfect people for the Australians, as for Bourignon, are those that have (or possibly have maintained), both sexes.

Sadeur is discussed, according to Bayle, in order to 'give a supplement to the chimerical fancies of Antoinette Bourignon'.[24] Returning to the 'Adam' article, 'Sadeur' is linked here by Bayle, claiming that 'the romantic Narrations of James Sadeur might as well be emply'd for that Purpose'.[25] What purpose this is remains confused. If Bayle means the purpose of describing hermaphrodites in general, his lack of references to historical hermaphrodites, say from medical treatises, makes little sense. If we believe he is interested in claiming Sadeur may support Bourignon's notion of a prelapsarian hermaphrodite, then intriguing options open for how Bayle is connecting these articles.

If this is the case, there is something necessarily connected between the description of Australia and the description of the Edenic paradise. Even though both remain mythological accounts, the situating of Australia in the 'real world' prompts speculation on human origins and the gravity of the fall. This seems to be the impetus behind the following comment in 'Sadeur':

> the inhabitants of Terra Australis are of Mrs Bourignon's opinion; and one would be apt to think that James Sadeur, whoever he was, designed to insinuate that those people are not descended from Adam, but from an androgyne, who did not fall, as Adam did, from his state of innocence. This might be a pretty good device to impose upon the censors of books, and remove the difficulties of a licence, if one had a mind to try the success of a pre-[A]damitical System.[26]

These fascinating remarks indicate that Bayle, though recognizing the tale as fictional, sees the potential for it *theologically*. By detaching the Edenic

24 Art. 'Sadeur'. See also Ferguson, 'L'Hermaphrodite sceptique'.
25 Art. 'Adam'.
26 Art. 'Sadeur'.

paradise from a description of the entirety of the human race and postulating the existence of beings which have maintained a pre-Adamic state (despite Bayle himself denying that this pre-Adamic state was hermaphroditic), one could defend views that isolate the Adam story to the origins of a segment of humanity, usually the Jewish nation. Bayle mentions Isaac La Peyrère by name in the 'Sadeur' article as one who may have benefitted from endorsing such a position. La Peyrère infamously wrote *Prae-Adamitae* in 1641 arguing that there were people before Adam and that the biblical prehistory is of a localized nature.

Bayle's article about La Peyrère is sparse, but it seems likely Bayle agreed with his sentiments if not his conclusions. According to Richard Popkin, La Peyrère claimed that 'as long as he was a Calvinist, he had to accept the pre-Adamite theory, since it agreed better with right reason, the natural sense of Scripture, and his individual conscience'.[27] Not only did Bayle share his Calvinist perspective, those are the same three interpretive principles Bayle seeks to follow, as demonstrated most eloquently in the *Philosophical Commentary*. Bayle, ever open to challenging convention and continuing conversations, may have encouraged such challenges to traditional doctrines and interpretations, even if he did not accept them himself. In 'Sadeur' we see Bayle explicitly put forth the mythic hermaphrodite as a challenge to contemporary understandings of divine creation.

Salmacis

The final place where Bayle explores the hermaphroditic body in depth is the article 'Salmacis'. This article describes the mythological nymph recounted by Ovid who, in love with Hermaphroditus, son of Hermes and Aphrodite, threw herself upon him and asked the gods to be joined forever with him. The gods granted her request and they became one person with both sexes. Bayle connects this article with the previous hermaphroditic links and it continues the ongoing theme of retelling mythological stories within this web of articles. The remarks appended here do not bear on hermaphrodites in particular but have some intriguing comments about the falsity of solely ascribing aggression and tenderness to males and females respectively, each sex can be sexually passionate in different ways. Although Bayle does affirm that men are primarily the aggressors and women properly the resistors because the question concerns the resistance of the heart not the body

27 Popkin, *The History of Scepticism*, p. 226.

and 'belongs in justice to the sex, which exceeds the other in beauty, good air, and address'.[28] If women were the 'aggressors' in pursuing men, Bayle comically surmises there would be very little resistance at all. Thus the story is used to challenge gendered emotions in society, albeit too mildly for modern tastes. Strength is reframed as an attribute belonging to the female heart in its resistive capacity. Once again, however, even as a 'lesson' is learned from the tale of Salmacis, hermaphrodites remain described by Bayle only in the mythological sense.

The disrupting hermaphrodite

Bayle has a well-established reputation as a writer who enjoys subverting ingrained positions, especially religious thought. Though his motives are disputed and can be interpreted as fideistic or anti-religious, the fact that Bayle intentionally disrupts the status quo is indisputable. From positing a society of virtuous atheists to attacking the reputation of King David, Bayle challenges commonplace religious views through far-ranging sceptical inquiry.[29]

Most infamously this subversive manoeuvre takes place in the *Dictionnaire* articles of 'Manichees' and 'Paulicians', where Bayle suggests the problem of evil cannot be resolved. No rational answer can be provided for why evil persists in the presence of an omnipotent, omniscient and benevolent God. The only option for maintaining Christian belief is to have faith despite the insolubility of evil. It is in the irrational that faith persists. And curiously, it is in not providing an answer that the dialog remains open for how faith can persist despite evil. That traditional solutions to the problem of evil are undermined is clear, the reader must decide whether this is Bayle's destruction of religion or reliance on faith above dogma. The subversive element of Bayle's infamous discussions of evil is a principle employed in the inherent subversiveness of the hermaphrodite.

In constructing his web of hermaphrodites, Bayle shows an awareness of the history of the hermaphroditic figure as an image of satire and subversion most famously used in, loosely veiled, satirical descriptions of Henri III and his court in Thomas Artus's *L'Isle des hermaphrodites* (1605). Bayle mentions this work in 'Salmacis' and notes the satirical slant of Artus, making clear his own acknowledgment of the hermaphrodite potential to

28 Art. 'Salmacis', Rem. B.
29 Bayle, *Various Thoughts*; *Dictionnaire* art. 'David'.

challenge society. Kathleen Long succinctly describes the societal disruption the hermaphrodite figures saying, 'What seems to menace dogmatically ordered French society is the acceptance that there may be more than one perspective on any issue.'[30] The hostile French political climate was imaged by hermaphroditic figures in the seventeenth century. Within the contexts of Protestant/Catholic hostilities, the hermaphrodite offers a literal disputed body in which opposing natures coexist. While illustrating division within a body, the hermaphrodite could also be rendered positively as a location of toleration between dissenting positions. Naturally, whether such coexistence is indeed possible, both for the state and for the hermaphrodite, lingers behind such portrayals. If such an inquiring role is afforded the hermaphroditic figure, Bayle may be using it in a similar way to interrogate not the political state but the state of 'man'.

Without trying to overstate an argument from absence, I nevertheless want to circle back to the lack of historical referents to hermaphrodites within Bayle's remarks. Legal cases surrounding hermaphrodites in the seventeenth century would certainly have been known to Bayle and his meticulous marginal citation of historical details lead me to believe the absence of such citations in these hermaphroditic articles is significant. This is not to say that the absence of hermaphroditic legal cases is part of some masterful clandestine argument but only the more obvious recognition that Bayle's mind may simply have been on other matters as he was crafting these remarks.

I believe this absence of concrete references serves well to highlight the liminality of the hermaphroditic body. While readers would be aware of historical referents for hermaphrodite bodies, locating them in myth emphasizes the disrupting element of the hermaphroditic figure.

The mythical location of Bayle's hermaphrodites is a stark contrast to Bayle's writings on supernatural signs and wonders in his *Pensées diverses* (1682). Here, the philosopher writes against those who would see natural phenomena, particularly comets, as divine signs signalling doom or fortune.[31] Scholars debate the degree to which this concern was legitimate in Bayle's time and perhaps his larger point was to challenge the acceptance of religious views based on the opinions of others, as when a 'sign' is determined. Nevertheless a rejection of the human ability to pinpoint and locate the supernatural in the world remains from this early writing throughout Bayle's work. The supernatural may not be wholly disqualified, but our ability to learn of the divine is minimal, and only through revelation if at

30 Long, *Hermaphrodites*, p. 220.
31 Daston and Park, *Wonders*, p. 252.

all. While Bayle's hermaphrodites do not exist as signs within the natural world, his restriction of them to a mythic category despite awareness of the hermaphroditic medical treatise enforces the hermaphrodite as a useful and loaded concept for engaging sceptical and theological reflection.

Mythic, mystic monsters

For Antoinette Bourignon, it is not the hermaphroditic Adam which is the monster. Rather, after the entrance of sin into the world, men have become 'Monsters in Nature, divided into two imperfect Sexes'.[32] The human body becomes necessarily imperfect in having lost the perfected form's ability to procreate alone. Although this aspect of Bourignon's thought is unexplored by Bayle it seems likely that, for Bourignon, part of the image of God in created man was the ability to self-create. After the Fall, procreation can only be done in tandem, the image of God has been marred. Of interest is the resituating of the elements of the Creation story. The splitting of Adam and Eve is pre-Fall in the traditional understanding. Yet for Bourignon, the creation of these sexed 'Monsters of Nature' is a result *of* the Fall. This is indeed puzzling and difficult to reconcile given her insistence on using the Fall narrative in a traditional way to explain the entrance of sin into the world.

The changing and conflicting accounts of the early modern hermaphrodite show a figure that could stand in as a variety of challenges to the status quo. Bourignon's alchemic figuring of the hermaphroditic Adam as perfect humanity runs counter to the hermaphrodite as 'confusion' or of an imperfect male/female.[33] In the hermaphroditic Adam, elements seen as counter to each other in the 'real' world are evidenced as harmonized. For the alchemical tradition this is, of course, the great goal, transmutation of contradictories into a different substance.[34] Still, in this striving for a more perfect state with the hermaphroditic figure functioning as ideal, everyday experience would have to be reordered and acknowledged as imperfect. The hermaphrodite, whether perfected or marred humanity, is a point of subversion, a disruption of order.[35]

It is possible this procreation aspect is another reason why Bayle declines to speak of historical accounts of real hermaphrodites. Bayle surely

32 Art. 'Adam', Rem. G.

33 See Long, *Hermaphrodites*, p. 243.

34 DeVun, 'The Jesus Hermaphrodite', pp. 194-195.

35 Gilbert, *Early Modern Hermaphrodites*, pp. 1-3.

understands that 'hermaphrodite' is used in two different ways in the period: 1) those who can procreate asexually, as Bourignon's Adam, and 2) people born with both sexual organs, intersexed. The first term remains discussed in medical treatises as a 'perfect' hermaphrodite with various degrees of scepticism over the very possibility of such a body existing. If Bayle is only interested in discussing and disproving the first example and is restricting his usage of hermaphrodite to this case, the absences of historical referents are understandable.

Bayle puts forward a fairly negative opinion of Antoinette Bourignon.[36] However, while mocking many elements of her life and her 'enthusiasm' or unrestrained prophetic behaviour, Bayle is much kinder to Bourignon than to those prophets he feels promote dangerous behaviour within the *Dictionnaire*. Perhaps he views her as an honest, but misguided person. One of the first statements related about Bourignon is that 'she knew already that Christians did not live according to their Principles'.[37] As Bayle makes the same point himself in a number of locations, notably within the *Pensées diverses* and the article 'Mahomet' of the *Dictionnaire*, he likely has a favourable view of Bourignon's rebellion from 'orthodoxy' even if Bayle may disagree with her particular doctrinal conclusions. Both Bayle and Bourignon are critical of the Christian culture of their time. The main text of the article devoted to Bourignon has Bayle straightforwardly convey that '[s]he learnt a great many particular things by Revelation; and it was then that she had the Visions which I spoke of in the Remarks of the Article ADAM.'[38] That this statement should be presented without critical judgement in the main text is at first perhaps not so surprising for Bayle devotes his lengthy remarks to particular notes on issues within articles. And yet, as an historical and critical dictionary, his stated purpose was to correct misunderstandings about people, places and things. If he thought Bourignon was particularly fraudulent, we should expect to see some mention of it in the main body.

One intriguing dimension of Bayle's discussion of the hermaphroditic Adam is to consider the exposure Bayle himself had to these ideas and his choosing Bourignon's remarks as a jumping off point. The androgynous Adam interpretation, sometimes devoid of self-reproductive ability, has a

36 For critique of Bayle's reading and Bourignon's lasting image, see De Baar, 'Conflicting Discourses'. De Baar criticizes Bayle for his 'misogynist' treatment of Bourignon. While this may an appropriate charge, Bayle's concerns with Bourignon seem to stem primarily from his fear of enthusiasm and Bayle's critique of Bourignon is similar to his other enthusiastic targets in the *Dictionnaire*.

37 Art. 'Bourignon', Rem. A.

38 Art. 'Bourignon'.

long history within rabbinic interpretation. Elliot Wolfson explains that although this androgynous reading has a long history, it often remained androcentric and did not privilege the hermaphroditic Adam.[39] That is, Adam had to be separated into Adam and Eve in order to be completed as God intended. Procreation was not, contra Bourignon, possible in the androgynous state. And yet, Wolfson notes, this maintains an androcentric interpretation of human origins. It is the restoration *to* the male of the female through sexual union that makes them 'one flesh' once more. The superiority of the male is affirmed in the traditional androgyne readings.[40] Bourignon's interpretation stands apart from these in emphasizing the equality of the sexes. They are imperfect apart, and need each other. Both were once perfect when they were located within one being.

While it would be overly speculative to assign any sort of particular favour towards kabbalistic thinking to Bayle, it is not out of place to acknowledge that Bayle had been exposed to these ideas through the Furly circle. The Quaker Benjamin Furly held gatherings for his diverse circle of friends and colleagues at his home in Rotterdam.[41] The Furly circle included the great minds of John Locke and Jean Leclerc as well as hosting appearances from the Christian kabbalist Francis Mercury van Helmont. The one appearance of Benjamin Furly's name within Bayle's *Dictionnaire* comes as a citation within the 'Bourignon' article previously discussed. Bayle draws on Furly to place a degree of separation between Quakers, like Furly, and the Quietist mysticism of Bourignon which, according to Furly, contains contradictions and presumably steps far beyond the limits of acceptable Christian beliefs. Within Furly's library, which Bayle had access to, is found the works of Bourignon as well as Van Helmont, Jacob Boehme's *Mysterium Magnum* and more explicitly kabbalistic sources.[42]

Van Helmont and Antoinette Bourignon shared the insights of the mystic Jacob Boehme (1575-1624), being different branches of the lineage of his thought. Within Boehme's writings one finds similarly strange views of Adam and odd interpretations of human origins drawing from kabbalistic thought. Boehme, like Bourignon later, wrote of a hermaphroditic Adam who could reproduce internally, the male and female 'Tinctures' mixing together in a union spurred by directing one's thoughts and love towards the divine.[43]

39 Wolfson, 'Bifurcating the Androgyne', p. 102.

40 Ibid.

41 See the collection of papers on Furly brought together by Sarah Hutton for more on this impactful meeting place of great minds. Hutton, *Benjamin Furly*.

42 *Bibliotheca Furliana*.

43 Almond, *Adam and Eve*, p. 176; Boehme, *Mysterium Magnum*, 19.8.

Yet for Boehme, the separation of Adam and Eve comes about through Adam's lusting after the carnality of the beasts.[44] The two are divinely separated and granted sexual organs in order to fulfil this sinful lust. Boehme differs from Bourignon in the focus of the Fall, being for Boehme a depiction of the nature of reality and Bourignon operating closer to orthodoxy in the Fall emerging from human action. However, in both accounts the separation of Adam and Eve from one, dual-sexed person comes about due to sin and God's granting of their sinful desires. More importantly, it is clear from Boehme's account that this involves a radically different chronology of the Genesis story, predating the seduction of Eve.

The mystic thought associated with Bourignon and her like carries a tendency to challenge and reread creation narratives for various ends. In engaging the hermaphrodite as a figure to enter these primordial stories Bayle takes up these challenges for his own ends. The hermaphrodite offers a both/and unresolved image, a sceptical suspension of judgement, to inhabit talk of origins, and with it foundational theological doctrine. The Behmist tales of Adam show how familiar stories can be dislodged and reread. I believe Bayle's repeated connections of hermaphroditic figures to mythic origin stories offer an ongoing challenge, or reappraisal, of the original state of humanity. Particularly, the questions of whether the hermaphrodite is a body marred by sin or perfectly formed linger behind all accounts and bring along the question of how sin has damaged humanity. Bayle, true to form, offers no solution, but through the hermaphroditic web directs readers of the 'Adam' article and related networks towards questions of the role of original sin in marring humanity.

Opening questions: A Baylean conclusion

The language of the monstrous prompted this investigation into Bayle's thought concerning the impact of sin on the human body. The popularity of travel literature for this period indicates why Bayle has moved away from his earlier rejection of popular curiosities and devotes entire articles to extravagant reports: this stuff sells. People were fascinated by accounts of faraway lands with terrible creatures and fantastical savages. The 'savage' body is a focusing rod of erotic discussion. The performative prudence of European civilization is permitted to be stripped away in these frank discussions. Much the same applies for stories of the paradisal state of humanity. Adam and Eve, fruitful

44 Boehme, *Mysterium Magnum*, 19.25.

and multiplying, are necessarily erotic in nature. Bayle links these two discussions around the point of hermaphrodism. Through provoking remarks and explicit cross-references, Bayle guarantees his readers are as engaged as he is.

The question is left provokingly open as to whether the joined hermaphroditic body is more perfect than a sexually divided humanity.[45] As mentioned, Bayle does not stress this point to the end of endorsing such mystical readings but uses them to guide more pressing questions about how a paradisal human would appear. Happy to leave his readers with more questions than answers, Bayle nevertheless complicates ongoing debates on sin by indicating that different positions, such as a pre-Adamite hypothesis, offer different benefits to our theological understandings. It is not only the ambiguity of the hermaphrodite which is subversive but the back and forth shifts between the interpretation of the figure as idyllic humanity and deformed monster. Ever the sceptic, what the *real* answer may be is unknown, but perhaps we can retrieve a paradisal state by functioning as undivided bodies in our suspension of judgement on insoluble matters.

Bayle's use of the hermaphrodite to direct questions of theological anthropology demonstrates the ongoing importance of the 'monster' figure. At its most reduced form Christian theology claims that what the human is now is not what it should be or 'was'. Monstrous figures snap our attention to this distortion of creation regardless of whether they point to further distortion of humanity, as early modern discussions of the sinful nature of man and modern monster movies tend, or gesture to an original state, as Bayle's hermaphrodites.

Works Cited

Primary Sources

Bayle, Pierre, *The Dictionary Historical and Critical of Mr Peter Bayle*, trans. P. Desmaizeaux, 2nd ed. (London: Knapton et al., 1734).

Bayle, Pierre, *A Philosophical Commentary on These Words of the Gospel, Luke XIV. 23. Compel Them to Come in, That My House May Be Full. In Four Parts.* 2 vols (London: J. Darby, 1708), new ed. J. Kilcullen and C. Kukathas (Indianapolis: Liberty Fund, 2005).

45 Bayle draws reference to Plato's discussion (in the *Symposium*, 189e-193c of the perfect hermaphrodite throughout these articles, most notably 'Adam', Rem. F, and 'Sadeur', Rem. F. These discussions are largely explanatory, providing the reader with the description of Plato's hermaphrodites. The mythic context is sustained.

Bayle, Pierre, *Various Thoughts on the Occasion of a Comet*, trans. Robert Bartlett (Albany: State University of New York Press, 2000).
Bibliotheca Furliana, sive catalogus librorum honoratiss. Et doctiss. Viri Benjamin Furly, inter quos excellunt bibliorum editiones, mystici, libri proprii cujuscumque sectae christianae, et manuscripti membranei (Rotterdam: Fritsch et Bohm, 1714).
Boehme, Jacob, *Mysterium Magnum: Or, An Exposition of the First Book of Moses Called Genesis* (London, 1654).
Plato. *Plato in Twelve Volumes,* Vol. 9 trans. Harold N. Fowler. (Cambridge, MA, Harvard University Press; London, William Heinemann Ltd. 1925) Perseus Digital Library. http://www.perseus.tufts.edu/hopper/text?doc=Perseus%3Atext%3A1999.01.0174%3Atext%3DSym. (Accessed October 10, 2020).

Secondary Sources

Almond, Philip C., *Adam and Eve in Seventeenth-Century Thought* (Cambridge: Cambridge University Press, 1999).
Bost, Hubert, 'Bible et fables: "Adam" et "Ève" dans le *Dictionnaire historique et critique* de Bayle', in *Adam et Ève et la pensée des Lumières: entre fondement du droit et questionnement du mythe*, ed. Gabriele Vickermann-Ribémont (Clermont-Ferrand: Presses universitaires Blaise Pascal, 2014), pp. 53-73.
Daston, Lorraine, and Katharine Park, 'The Hermaphrodite and the Orders of Nature: Sexual Ambiguity in Early Modern France', *GLQ: A Journal of Lesbian and Gay Studies* 1 (1995), pp. 419-438.
Daston, Lorraine, and Katharine Park, *Wonders and the Order of Nature, 1150-1750* (New York: Zone Books, 1998).
De Baar, Mirjam, 'Conflicting Discourses on Female Dissent in the Early Modern Period: The Case of Antoinette Bourignon (1616-1680)', *L'Atelier du Centre de recherches historiques*, 4 September 2009. http://journals.openedition.org/acrh/1399; DOI: 10.4000/acrh.1399 (accessed 25 October 2018).
DeVun, Leah, 'Heavenly Hermaphrodites: Sexual Difference at the Beginning and End of Time' *Postmedieval: A Journal of Medieval Cultural Studies* 9, no. 2 (2018), pp. 132-146.
DeVun, Leah, 'The Jesus Hermaphrodite: Science and Sex Difference in Premodern Europe' *Journal of the History of Ideas* 69, no. 2 (2008), pp. 193-218.
Ferguson, Gary, 'L'Hermaphrodite sceptique: *La Terre Australe connue* de Gabriel de Foigny', in *L'Hermaphrodite de la Renaissance aux Lumières*, ed. Marianne Closson (Paris: Classiques Garnier, 2013), pp. 257-279.
Gilbert, Ruth, *Early Modern Hermaphrodites: Sex and Other Stories* (New York: Palgrave, 2002).

Graille, Patrick, *Les Hermaphrodites aux XVIIe et XVIIIe siècles* (Paris: Les Belles Lettres, 2001).
Hutton, Sarah, ed., *Benjamin Furly 1646-1714: A Quaker Merchant and His Milieu* (Firenze: L.S. Olschki, 2007).
Labrousse, Elisabeth, *Bayle* (Oxford: Oxford University Press, 1983).
Laqueur, Thomas, *Making Sex: Body and Gender from the Greeks to Freud* (Cambridge, MA: Harvard University Press, 1992).
Lennon, Thomas M., and Michael Hickson, 'Pierre Bayle', *The Stanford Encyclopedia of Philosophy* (Winter 2017 Edition), ed. Edward N. Zalta. https://plato.stanford.edu/archives/win2017/entries/bayle/ (accessed 3 June 2020).
Long, Kathleen P., 'From Monstrosity to Postnormality: Montaigne, Canguilhem, Foucault', in *Monstrosity, Disability, and the Posthuman in the Medieval and Early Modern World*, ed. Richard H. Godden and Asa Simon Mittman (New York: Palgrave Macmillan, 2019), pp. 35-61.
Long, Kathleen P., *Hermaphrodites in Renaissance Europe* (Aldershot: Ashgate, 2006).
Park, Katharine, and Lorraine J. Daston, 'Unnatural Conceptions: The Study of Monsters in Sixteenth- and Seventeenth-Century France and England', *Past and Present* 92, no. 1 (1981), pp. 20-54.
Popkin, Richard, *The History of Scepticism: From Savonarola to Bayle* (Oxford: Oxford University Press, 2003).
Van der Lugt, Mara, *Bayle, Jurieu, and the* Dictionnaire Historique et Critique (Oxford: Oxford University Press, 2016).
Van Lieshout, H.H.M., *The Making of Pierre Bayle's* Dictionnaire Historique et Critique, trans. Lynne Richards (Amsterdam: APA-Holland University Press, 2001).
Wolfson, Elliot R., 'Bifurcating the Androgyne and Engendering Sin: A Zoharic Reading of Gen 1-3', in *Hidden Truths from Eden: Esoteric Readings of Genesis 1-3*, ed. Caroline Vander Stichele and Susanne Scholz (Atlanta: SBL Press, 2014), pp. 83-115.

About the Author

Parker Cotton is a PhD candidate in theology at Wycliffe College, University of Toronto. His academic interests are focused on toleration and scriptural interpretation of the early modern period. His dissertation examines Pierre Bayle's use of scripture in arguments for religious toleration.

6. An Education: Johannes Schefferus and the Prodigious Son of a Fisherman[1]

Maja Bondestam

Abstract

In this essay, the value of monsters and prodigies is examined in relation to seventeenth-century learned reflection and the German-Swedish intellectual Johannes Schefferus. Earlier research on the positive meaning of wonders has highlighted the Augustinian tradition of reading prodigious bodies as reminders of God's presence. Schefferus himself emphasized a cultural heritage in which strange and thought-provoking bodies were considered educational and morally enhancing. A monstrous birth and a boy with a prodigious appearance thus functioned as a teacher of virtue, a guiding example and an object of contemplation. For Schefferus, this pedagogical and moral potential was the reason why such a body should be displayed and remembered through museums, histories, books and images.

Keywords: prodigies, monstrous births, seventeenth century, Sweden, knowledge, virtue

In 1668, a boy with a so-called prodigious appearance was born in Norrtälje, north of Stockholm, and according to present witnesses, he deviated in a number of ways from the expected shape and size of a newborn child. We meet this son of a fisherman in a manuscript wherein the renowned intellectual Johannes Schefferus, in line with older prodigy tales, presented a collection of exceptional, unique and thought-provoking bodies, things and phenomena.[2]

1 This chapter was written as a part of the research programme *Medicine at the borders of life: Fetal research and the emergence of ethical controversy in Sweden*, supported by the Swedish Research Council (Dnr 2014–1749).

2 Schefferus, 'Variae historiae', chap. IV. My accounts and quotations from the manuscript in this essay are based upon a forthcoming translation from the Latin by Anna Fredriksson, PhD,

Bondestam, M. (ed.), *Exceptional Bodies in Early Modern Culture: Concepts of Monstrosity before the Advent of the Normal*. Taylor & Francis Group, 2020
DOI 10.5117/9789463721745_CH06

Schefferus was educated in Strassburg, Leiden and Switzerland and in 1648, Queen Christina invited him to Sweden. Here he got a professorship in rhetoric and politics at Uppsala University and became active in a number of fields, not least as a philologist and historian. This chapter examines Schefferus's representations and mediations on rare, astonishing and unexpected bodies, births and objects, and discusses their value. The social aspects of knowledge are in focus and I try to situate the movements, practices and materiality of Schefferus's exceptional collection. How did it come about, for whom was it compiled and how was knowledge of prodigies and monsters consumed in seventeenth-century Sweden? Throughout the essay, I have a local starting point but hope to write a history with broad significance.[3]

The boy in Norrtälje was presented in the manuscript together with a number of other remarkable bodies and things, such as the monster from the parish of Lillebered, near Västerås, which was born right beside the village council's official meeting place. There was also a description of a large stone found in the bladder of a man from Nürnberg and shown to Schefferus when he lived in Strassburg, and drawings of an old golden ring with an intriguing decoration, thought to have been owned by Bridget of Sweden, the mystic and saint from the fourteenth century. Schefferus also described a mine in which those who entered died, and an Englishman with no arms and very short feet, who displayed himself for money in the surroundings of Uppsala. He pictured a woman who became grey-haired in her youth and then blonde again when she died many years later; a maid who once met with what was thought to be the evil spirit of the water, the Neck; and a stalk of wheat that flowered twice in one season. In nine chapters under the title 'Variae historiae', Schefferus described these exceptional singularities, which he had either experienced first-hand or was told about by some truthful person, such as Ursula Tamm, known in Uppsala for her veracious perception. Tamm was married to Schefferus's colleague and close friend Johannes Loccenius, and was the one who told him about the woman with unexpected hair colour in relation to her age.[4]

In this essay, I want to contribute to the history of monsters and portents, their value and meaning, in medicine and learned reflection. I examine Schefferus's collections of exceptional bodies, things and phenomena and focus on his search for knowledge and virtue in the seventeenth century. The point I want to make is that prodigious bodies in the positive Augustinian

Uppsala University Library.

3 Secord, 'Knowledge in Transit', pp. 655-656, 662-664, 668.

4 Schefferus, 'Variae historiae', chaps I-VIII.

tradition not only connected to wonders through the emotion evoked by them, by the praising of wonders as a testimony of their omnipotent creator, or by an intellectual tradition elaborated from high medieval European writings about a human appetite for the rare, novel and strange.[5] A collection of prodigious bodies, things and phenomena could, as I will show, also educate and morally edify the beholder. Monsters, at least from the perspective of Schefferus, made people better persons, heightened their virtue and functioned as illuminating examples and guiding images.

Prodigies and monsters in seventeenth-century Sweden

The words used for describing exceptional bodies in early modern Swedish culture reveal strong feelings of excitement. In folk belief and mythology the terms *monster*, *wonder* and *portent* have been used metaphorically about animalistic beings with frightening appearances, and about bodies and things deviating from all expectations in shape, size and attributes. Failure, wonder and an ominous symbolism have been associated with monsters, and they have been interpreted as negations of right and proper beings.[6] In the seventeenth century satyrs and banshees, evil spirits and humanlike animals, invoked in judicial procedures and trials regarding bestiality and demonic sexuality, could bring to mind the carnal and animate dimensions of human nature.[7]

The word *prodigious* (*prodigiös*) has been used in the Swedish language since at least 1633 as a synonym for something odd, unnatural, fantastic or unheard of, while a prodigy (*prodigium*) was a portent, a wonder or an odd occurrence.[8] A dissertation about portents defended at Uppsala University in 1676 explained that a prodigious thing was something that went beyond the ordinary course of events in nature, something revealed for us, and by God's special permission notifying people of future events.[9] Dictionaries also indicate that the word *monster* in early modern Swedish was used as a synonym for *wonder*, *deformed person*, *portent* and *beast*.[10]

5 Daston and Park, *Wonders*, pp. 21, 76; Bates, *Emblematic Monsters*, pp. 11-12, 14, 21-22, 24-25.

6 *Ordbok över svenska språket*, XVII, column M 1321, under *monster*; *Nationalencyklopedins ordbok*, II, p. 398; *Nordisk familjebok*, XI, p. 271.

7 Liliequist, *Brott, synd och straff*, pp. 89-167; Häll, *Skogsrået, näcken och djävulen*, pp. 86-89.

8 *Ordbok över svenska språket*, XX, column P 1945, under *prodigiös*.

9 Columbus and Dwan, *Dissertatio academica*, chaps I, III.

10 Hellquist, *Svensk etymologisk ordbok*, p. 483; *Ordbok över svenska språket*, XVII, column M 1321, under *monster*; Dalin, *Ordbok öfver svenska språket*, II, p. 105.

In 'Variae historiae', Schefferus indicated that prodigies and monsters were not only bad and frightening omens, creatures contrary to nature and divine will or signs of disapproval sent by God. They could also bring virtue and knowledge, which reminds us of the productive nature of the monster in Rosemary Moore's discussion of fugitive sheets and the monstrous Medusa figure.[11] Monsters and prodigies had, as we will see, a remarkable and outstanding ability to arouse surprise and admiration, remind people of something specific and encourage their moral advancement. In European elite culture, at the courts, in trade and travel, and among collectors, scholars, physicians and apothecaries, a similar capacity was attached to rare and extraordinary natural objects. Cabinets of curiosities or *Kunst- und Wunderkammern* were, as Krzysztof Pomian writes, part of a tradition wherein strange and exceptional natural specimens were highly valued in the sixteenth and seventeenth centuries.[12] Lorraine Daston and Katharine Park have shown that wonders, such as precious, exotic and rare animals, plants and minerals in the same period were appreciated, collected and exchanged because they illustrated a playfulness, sensibility, creativity and variability in nature.[13] Paula Findlen and Camilla Mordhorst claim that collectors of natural objects in the fifteenth, sixteenth and seventeenth centuries paid attention to and cared for the deviating, incomprehensible and particular case. Here, something specific and unexpected could facilitate the understanding of nature, explain the inexplicable and display recurrent principles of irregularity.[14]

Monstrous births in fifteenth- and sixteenth-century Europe were also part of a popular genre of broadsheets, ballads, pamphlets and advertisements in which every new body was pictured and placed in a certain context; in all their specificity, these accounts offered important insights and symbols to contemplate and decode. Alan W. Bates claims that the use of monsters as emblems and symbols in such prints puts more importance on the individual case, its form, character and distinct connection to time and space, than did medical and natural philosophical works at the time.[15]

In relation to the monster category in early modern elite culture, as described by Pomian, Daston, Park, Findlen, Mordhorst and Bates, and in what we today call England, Italy, Germany, France and Denmark, the

11 Moore, 'Monsters and the Maternal Imagination', in this volume.

12 Pomian, *Collectors and Curiosities*, pp. 45-47, 64.

13 Daston and Park, *Wonders*, pp. 146-172, 190-191, 193-201, 215-253.

14 Findlen, *Possessing Nature*, pp. 48-101; Mordhorst, *Genstandsfortællinger*, pp. 143-200.

15 Bates, *Emblematic Monsters*, p. 57.

Swedish context differs in a number of ways. I have only found one text written in Swedish of the kind Bates describes, a broadsheet detailing the characteristics and history of a particular monstrous birth or individual, and it is a translation.[16] Neither were there in seventeenth-century Sweden any scientific journals that could pick up the structure of the old broadsheet, the case study with its typical introduction, description of a particular case and final discussion.[17] Members of the Swedish court did not collect natural curiosities before the eighteenth century, although gifts and exchanges existed earlier and reached the royal palaces and treasure chambers, as they did around Europe.[18]

At Swedish universities in the second half of the seventeenth century, monsters and prodigies were the subject of a couple of dissertations. In Uppsala, Åbo, Greifswald, Dorpat and Lund, professors and students were writing and defending a great number of dissertations on specific topics, and on rare occasions monsters and prodigies were discussed. Such bodies, things and phenomena in the material world were approached a bit reluctantly, above all transformed into abstractions and concepts to be defined or treated as accidental deviations from the usual habits of nature. One author defended his choice of subject by announcing his ambition to explain for a wider audience that such formations were natural and had nothing to do with trolls or dark powers of some kind.[19]

Guiding images

Johannes Schefferus was a leading intellectual in the seventeenth century, a German-Swedish scholar in the humanities and a professor in political science at Uppsala University. Educated in Strassburg, Leiden, Amsterdam and Copenhagen, he came to Sweden in 1648 and started up pioneering work in a number of fields, as a linguistic researcher, literary historian, archaeologist, and historian. Above all, he is known for the work *Lapponia*, written to extend contemporary knowledge of Laplanders, and to dismiss

16 *En kort Berättelse.*

17 There was a desire among renowned physicians and natural historians in the late seventeenth century to start a scientific academy in accordance with foreign models, probably the Royal Society of London. Lindroth, 'Collegium medicum'.

18 Löwegren, *Naturaliekabinett i Sverige*, pp. 48-53.

19 Thauvonius and Gyllenius, *Disputatio physica inauguralis*; Weiser and Jacobi, *Disputatio physica*.

the rumour of their witchcraft as an explanation for the Swedes' great success on the battlefield.[20]

Schefferus published extensively during his career, mostly abroad because of bad printing conditions in Sweden. When he died in 1679, a number of his works were still in manuscript, and colleagues around Europe tried without success to have them printed.[21] 'Variae historiae' is one such manuscript, now kept at Uppsala University Library. It is written in Latin and represents a wonderful collection of unique bodies, things and phenomena, of which a few were illustrated by Schefferus, who was a skilled draughtsman. The wonders in the manuscript have a lot in common with ancient accounts of natural wonders and sketches of astonishing lives. It is full of surprises, strange objects and various singularities, inviting the reader to ponder contrasts between the expected and unexpected courses of nature. It is worth mentioning that in the 1640s Schefferus worked on an edition of the Roman author Claudius Aelianus's *Varia historia*, which probably inspired the title of his manuscript.[22]

Among Schefferus's notes and drawings is a description of the above-mentioned fisherman's son, born in Norrtälje on 12 April 1668, who had a prodigious appearance and deviated from the expected shape, size and attributes of a newborn in a number of ways. Schefferus informed the reader that the boy's head had an enormous mass above the forehead, which was covered with hair. In addition, the left ear hung from the head and resembled the ear of a calf, while the left hand looked like a foot and only had four fingers. A number of fundamental categories, which would be expected to remain clearly separate, were mixed and turned upside down in this boy. The usually obvious distinction between infant and adult was disrupted by the big head, the upper and the lower parts of the body were mixed, and so were human and animal attributes. The father, Erik Martinsson, wanted to keep his son's birth a secret and arranged for him to be buried immediately. However, the rumour of the boy's existence spread quickly, and Schefferus mentions how some officials (*magistratus*) arranged for the dead boy to be dug up, after which they inspected and drew pictures of him. The enormous head was opened up with a little knife, and a divided skull, each part of which was as big as that of a grown person, was found.[23]

20 Burius, 'Johannes Schefferus'.
21 Ibid., p. 519.
22 Aelianus, *Ailianou poikilēs historias*.
23 Schefferus, 'Variae historiae', chap. IV.

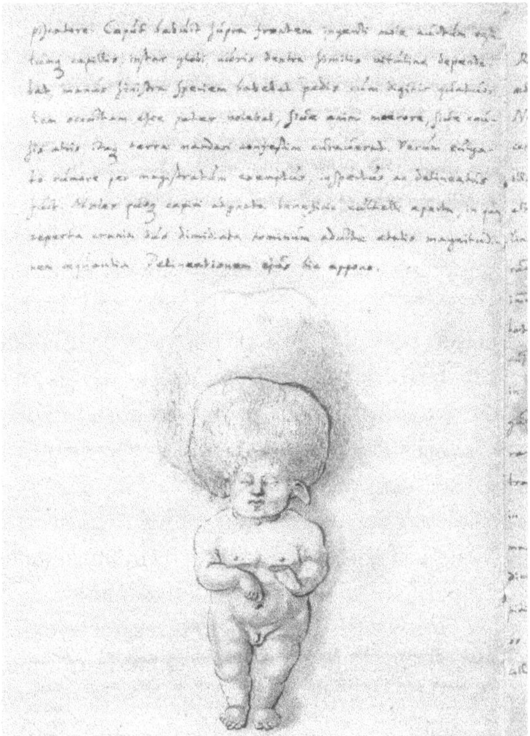

Figure 6.1. Johannes Schefferus, A boy with a so-called prodigious appearance. Drawing from Chapter IV of Johannes Schefferus, 'Variae historiae', 1670-1679, Uppsala University Library, MS X 292. Photograph: Uppsala University Library.

Schefferus does not tell us who the investigating officials were, but my guess is that they came from the Collegium Medicum, an institution of trained physicians founded in Stockholm in the middle of the seventeenth century. At this time, medically trained men got their educations outside the country, and when they got back to Sweden, they started to practice at the court, among the nobility, or in the army. There were also medical professorships and students in Uppsala, Lund and Åbo, and from the 1660s a fellowship of trained and chosen physicians in the Collegium Medicum. Queen Kristina's surgeon-in-ordinary, Grégoire François Du Rietz, initiated the Collegium. Du Rietz, brought in from France, was interested in founding an establishment where students could receive more formal education than either the self-taught physicians or the surgeons and bonesetters, who were educated in a mode of handiwork. In the 1640s, Uppsala University sent six medical students to Du Rietz, but teaching ceased after a couple of years, and no medical school was established during the rest of the century. Instead, Du

Rietz, together with three other physicians, founded the Collegium Medicum and in that way laid the foundation of an institution that would gain more and more privileges and some administrative authority as time went on.[24]

It is particularly interesting that doctors around the country were assigned to communicate to the Collegium 'what seemed to be rare and worth considering, in medicine or nature'.[25] Schefferus did not report any rare, prodigious or monstrous objects, bodies or phenomena to the Collegium Medicum, as far as I know, but could very well have done so. Singular and unique specimens were of certain interest for Schefferus, and 'Variae historiae' is a collection of precisely such objects. I have already mentioned the so-called monster from Lillebered, a small parish near Västerås, and just like the fisherman's son, this astonishing creature was born in 1668. The monstrous fetus, as Schefferus called it, was delivered by a sow and, in contrast to what is common for such animals, its head looked human. The birth took place outside a building where the farmers came together for legal consultations and was witnessed with great wonder by many people. Schefferus tells us that the top of the head and the neck had a number of wrinkled collops, just like a woman's bonnet. The creature was not unlike a piglet, but less bristly and instead covered with soft hair, like a newborn child, and the chest looked as if it was covered with a habergeon. Schefferus had seen piglets like this a long time before, but their heads had no outgrowths and looked like children's heads, although with more prominent noses and mouths. He drew a picture of the new offspring and presented it to the reader: 'But, behold, the look of the monster from Lillebered.'[26]

How could an animal deviate in this way from its usual appearance? Schefferus was far from sure but pointed out that this case reminded him of what the Roman fabulist Phaedrus, with reference to Aesop, had said about sheep with human heads. The ancient writer Aesop explained the peculiar mixed-up quality of such creatures by way of bestiality, although his major point was not to explain how they were generated but whom one should listen to when they appeared. When a creature with a human face was born, was it best to pay attention to someone who had learned by experience or to a soothsayer? According to Aesop, the experienced person

24 *Nordisk familjebok*, V, pp. 532-533; Hjelt, *Svenska och finska*, I, p. 17; Lindroth, 'Collegium medicum'.

25 'alla medici skola årligen eller vid förefallande lägenhet med syndico Collegii communicera hvad som rart och tänkvärdigt in re medica eller naturali mange förefalla'. Hjelt, *Svenska och finska*, II, p. 11.

26 'Sed en tibi monstri lillieberedensis speciem'. Schefferus, 'Variae historiae', chap. VIII.

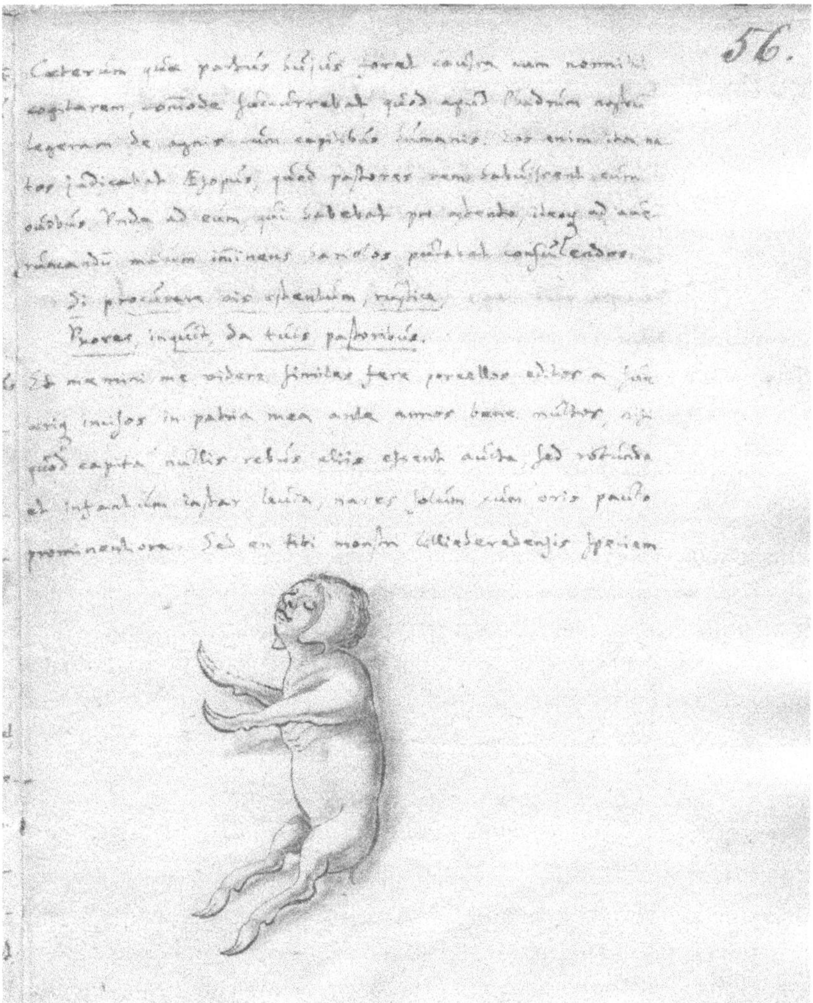

Figure 6.2. Johannes Schefferus, The monster from Lillebered. Drawing from Chapter VIII of Johannes Schefferus, 'Variae historiae', 1670-1679, Uppsala University Library, MS X 292. Photograph: Uppsala University Library.

was commonly believed to be a truer prophet than the soothsayer was, and his fable stresses the accuracy of this supposition:

> The ewes of a certain man who kept flocks gave birth to lambs with human heads. Being greatly alarmed at this prodigy and in deep dejection, he hastened to consult the soothsayers. One of them replied that this thing had reference to the owner's life, and that he must avert the danger by the sacrifice of a victim; another declared the meaning to be that his

> wife was an adulteress and his children spurious, but this omen could be dispelled at the cost of a larger sacrificial victim. Why say more? They all had different opinions and they increased the man's anxiety by the addition of greater anxiety. Aesop happened to be standing by, an old man of keen discernment, whom nature could never deceive; said he: 'If you wish to take proper measures to avert this portent, farmer, give wives to your shepherds.'[27]

Aristotle had explained that sexual intercourse between different species was infertile because of their different gestation periods, and according to Bates, there were seldom any insinuations in seventeenth-century dissertations that a mix of semen from human and animal preceded the birth of a monster.[28] Schefferus appears, however, to be more engaged with questions about empirical knowledge versus ominous signs than with explaining how monsters were produced. The reason why he referred to Aesop was, as I read him, to show whom one should listen to in the case of an extraordinary birth. The Latin words *monstrare* and *demonstro* mean 'to show', and the monster from Lillebered showed, like a good example or a fable, why people should find alternative interpreters to soothsayers and prognosticators, who focused on vague symbols, threats, sacrifices, victims, dangers and punishments.

The Swedes' most memorable examples

Schefferus's reference to Aesop might indicate a general scepticism towards portents and people's presumptions regarding God's power to produce direct warnings in nature. He criticized soothsayers and omens but saw guiding images as important parts of knowledge and virtue. In *Memorabilium Sueticae gentis exemplorum liber singularis*, or *Memorabilium liber* Schefferus presented a collection of extraordinary events, singular anecdotes and especially memorable examples in Swedish history. This was a textbook on politics and rhetoric, but the reader also got a chance to reflect upon (and gain virtue, knowledge and national self-esteem from) the most memorable examples in the history of the nation. Schefferus explained how remarkable signs in nature sometimes precede important changes in public life, unforeseen events and sad incidents.[29] Two such signs were seen when Birger

27 Phaedrus, 'Aesop and the Farmer', pp. 262-263.

28 Bates, *Emblematic Monsters*, pp. 118-119.

29 Schefferus, *En bok*, p. 45.

Magnusson became king of Sweden in the late thirteenth century. First, the water ceased to flow in a nearby river, and second, blood fell like rain over a castle in the river, called Ringstaholm. The Swedes were, according to Schefferus, bearers of many such memorable examples, a golden cultural heritage and a varied collection of stories, which, remembered in the right way, had the potential to make them a better people. *Memorabilium liber* is sometimes described as a minor classic of Swedish historical writing, and its stories have been passed down in textbooks and popular scientific presentations for centuries.[30]

Schefferus encouraged everyone to observe surprising and wonderful phenomena in their lives and in history and to memorize unusual, rare, unique and spectacular things. The anecdote about a nobleman who woke up in his coffin, buried, and had to eat his own flesh until he eventually died, is one such memory. It was valuable because those who were amazed by it were also connected to the divine will that maintains and rules the world.[31] Schefferus made no distinction in *Memorabilium liber* between noteworthy things in nature and in history; both should be displayed, admired, and remembered. In the same way as stories about kings and their deeds, rains of blood could be consulted for education and moral improvement but also, inspire specific actions. It is not far-fetched to suppose that Schefferus wanted to look at, draw pictures of, and think about exceptional bodies, things, and phenomena for similar reasons. He contributed to a cultural tradition wherein examples from history, nature, the Bible, and the ancient writers embraced singular and extraordinary events and accentuated their capacity to show people a certain pattern of living and how to increase their virtue.

The tradition of *exempla* is associated with ancient and medieval literary genres in which not only desirable, beautiful, and good scenarios in life were displayed, but also abominable and erroneous things for people to distance themselves from.[32] Lives, postures and actions of fictional and real people were portrayed to mimic or avoid, and the example itself was expected to teach the reader to see and draw conclusions. Texts delivered insights and assisted readers to make choices in their own terms. Reappearing images and examples were taken from nature, the Bible, and the ancient myths in a visual education, traceable into modern times.[33] Morality plays and allegorical figures in late medieval drama functioned as object lessons in how

30 Savin, 'Anekdoter om dygd', pp. 234, 241.

31 Ibid., pp. 235, 239, 244-245.

32 Bradley, 'Backgrounds', pp. 113-115.

33 Agrell, 'Att lära sig se', pp. 264-274.

to lead a good or bad life, but such unequivocal characters have continued to mediate religious, moral and political knowledge in more recent storytelling as well. Even in nineteenth-century legal texts, scientific and medical case studies, statistical reports, articles and notices in the press, individual lives were sometimes transformed into guiding examples. The morality play prescribed rather than recounted actions and mediated stereotyped role models and warnings to reflect upon.[34] Reinhart Koselleck has examined the notion of history as a teacher of life (*historia magistra vitae*) and how it was employed before the middle of the eighteenth century. Here, history appears as a collection of examples, including bad ones, and as a reservoir of multiplied experiences for readers to learn from and make their own. The examples were used instructively, as lessons for the future.[35]

In *Memorabilium liber* Schefferus compiled a number of events for the Swedish people to memorize and learn from, and 'Variae historiae' may have been written for similar reasons. The manuscript was never printed or widely read in the same way as *Memorabilium liber* but comprised a collection of astonishing bodies, rare natural objects and phenomena to be preserved as a cultural heritage.

The fisherman's son, the monster from Lillebered, the stone inside a man, Bridget of Sweden's ring, the maid's encounter with the Neck, the woman whose hair changed colour, the poisonous mine, the Englishman without arms and the doubly fruitful stalk of wheat should be memorized and contemplated to guide, educate and bring virtue. These odd and fascinating bodies and events deviated from the expected order of things and displayed mixed categories, species, purposes, ages, body parts and symbols. Characteristics of humans and animals, adults and children, young people and old, upper and lower limbs, could occasionally be found in the same body, which was thought-provoking. The Englishman wrote letters, played cards, ate soup and handled a needle and thread with his mouth – all to the spectators' wonder and delight, according to Schefferus.[36] The stone, found in the bladder of a man from Nürnberg after his death, and later displayed for Schefferus in Strassburg, was interesting because it altered the order of creation.[37] We would call it a gallstone or kidney stone, a precipitation of salts producing hard formations in the gall bladder or urinary tract, but Schefferus probably considered it a real stone, which made it wondrous. According

34 Ekström, *Dödens exempel*, pp. 13-15.

35 Koselleck, *Futures Past*, pp. 26-29.

36 Schefferus, 'Variae historiae', chap. V.

37 Ibid., chap. III.

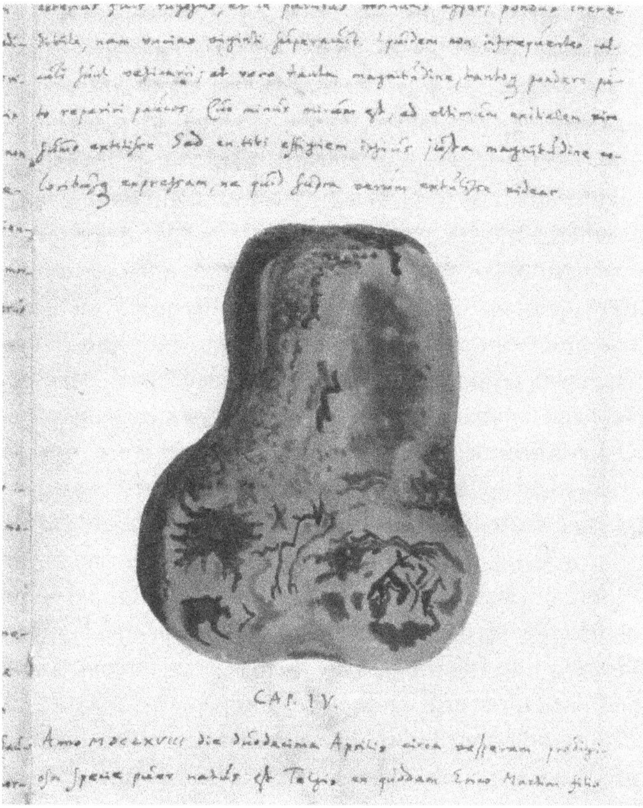

Figure 6.3. Johannes Schefferus, A large stone, found inside the bladder of a man. Drawing from Chapter III of Johannes Schefferus, 'Variae historiae', 1670-1679, Uppsala University Library, MS X 292. Photograph: Uppsala University Library.

to the Bible, God made mountains on the third day of creation, when he separated earth from water and before he created plants and animals. How was it possible, given this, to find stones inside humans and animals?[38] The stone raised fundamental questions about nature, history, God's agency, the creation and its inconsistencies. It would be a major contribution to human knowledge if these questions were answered.

Schefferus was not alone in emphasizing the importance of gallstones. On the contrary, such objects were held in high regard among the collecting physicians, botanists, mineralogists and librarians who from the second half of the century filled the cabinets with unexpected animals, plants, mineral, herbs, coins and other objects.[39] When the Swedish physician and collector

38 Fredriksson, 'A Changeable World', p. 29.
39 Bromelius, *Catalogus generalis*.

Magnus von Bromell died in 1731, he owned no fewer than twelve cabinets of natural specimens, some of which were sold, and others donated, to the court, the state, learned societies and universities.[40] The sixteenth-century physician Johannes Kentmann is also known to have collected stones found inside people's bodies. Different kinds of stones in brains, lungs, intestines, kidneys, and bladders apparently caused great amazement among both educated viewers and the broader public.[41]

The collecting of natural objects was a voluntary and time-consuming activity pursued by members of the European elite. To be the owner of a rare, paradoxical and wondrous object was a way to gain knowledge and prestige. In such collections, the remains of supposed mythical creatures, giants, satyrs and basilisks were placed next to fossils, gemstones, zoophytes and other animals, plants and minerals that were hard to systematize. How they had appeared in nature and why they transgressed prevailing orders of classification was far from clear. How could plants and animals be pictured and imitated deep inside mountains and in the hardest rocks? Where did the magnet's power to attract and repel come from? How could new species of animals emerge, having been unknown for centuries? The armadillo and the bird of paradise were not mentioned in ancient and medieval literature, and so the question was, What paradise had they originated from? If God had created them, they should have existed from the beginning and been described in some learned context over the centuries. Paula Findlen believes that the museums and collections of the fifteenth and sixteenth centuries tied together amazing, exotic and common natural specimens and represented nature as a continuum in which completely ordinary things could fill the gap between one paradox and the next. She describes the collecting of animals, plants and minerals as attempts to deal with the explosion of known things and bodies that was brought about by the wide dissemination of ancient texts, the extensive travel of the day, scientific discoveries and new forms of communication and exchange. Curiosity arose among Europeans towards distant cultures in these centuries and in the long run established an understanding of the *European order* as a relative, rather than absolute, measure of civilization.[42]

Beginning in the seventeenth century animals, plants, minerals and artefacts were also collected at Swedish universities and in private cabinets of

40 Löwegren, *Naturaliekabinett i Sverige*, p. 61.

41 Daston and Park, *Wonders*, p. 155.

42 Findlen, *Possessing Nature*, pp. 1-3.

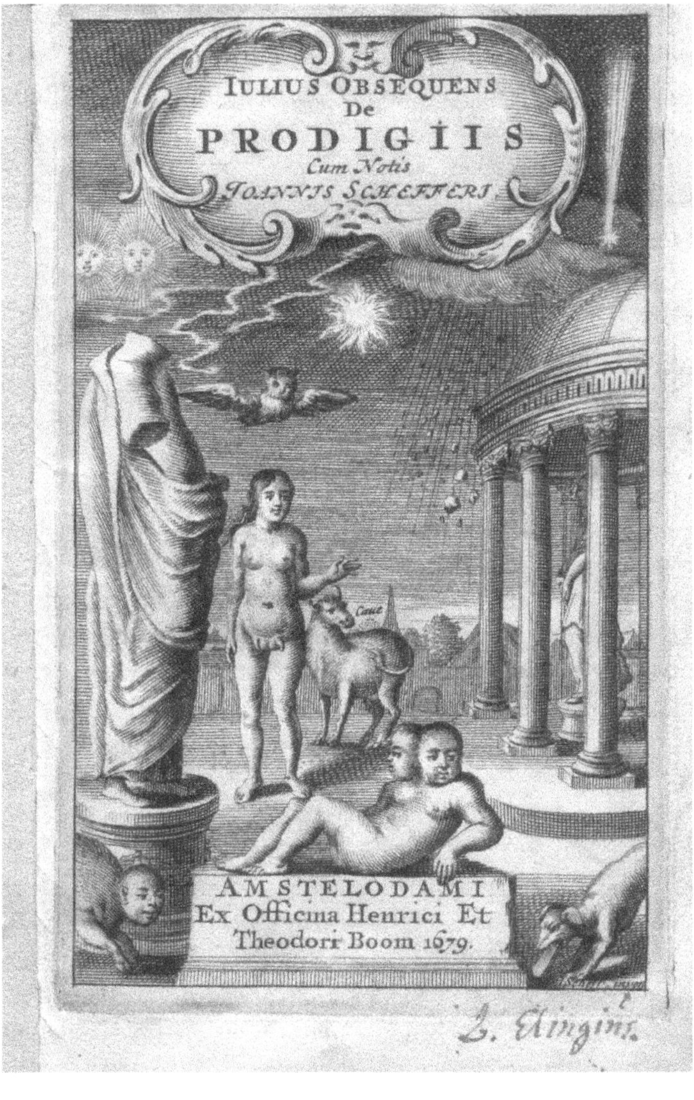

Figure 6.4. Frontispiece, Julius Obsequens and Conrad Lycosthenes, *Julii Obsequentis de prodigiis liber: cum annotationibus Joannis Schefferi [...] accedunt Conr. Lycosthenis supplementum Obsequentis; item librorum à Scheffero editorum index* (Stockholm, 1679). Photograph: Uppsala University Library.

curiosities. Schefferus had a museum of wonders that was a whole building, especially designed for the purpose, with a valuable collection of books, minerals, ethnographical objects, coins and other things that could be found in a *Kunst- or Wunderkammer* around this time. Masterpieces from both nature and culture, preferably mixed, seem to have attracted Schefferus, who mentions that, among other things in his museum, he had a hair threaded through a very tiny needle.[43] Museum Schefferianum has been called the first private cabinet of natural specimens in Sweden.[44]

Schefferus's editorial work was in a way like a collection of wondrous natural curiosities. In 1679, he republished the Roman writer Julius Obsequens's late antique book on wonders and portents, *De prodigiis liber*, extracted from Livy and describing unexpected elements of nature, history, and the cosmos in Rome between 249 BC and 12 BC. Obsequens's compendium was a collection of natural phenomena, interesting because of their singularity and meaning, and between 1508 and 1703 was published in eighteen different editions. Conrad Lycosthenes's *Prodigiorum liber* from 1552 is the most famous of these editions, and it supplemented Obsequens's compendium with new wonders. These were also included in Schefferus's edition, and the title page of his work shows a hermaphrodite, conjoined twins and an animal with a human face, as well as comets and other celestial phenomena. The book of wonders described exceptional and significant events, natural objects and notable phenomena, such as earthquakes and humans and animals from distant lands.[45] If Schefferus had the same motives for publishing a new edition of Obsequens's book as for collecting the most memorable examples of the Swedish people, we can imagine that he saw an opportunity to transform nature's most memorable examples and marvellous singularities into virtue and knowledge.

A disruptive history of monsters

In research on monsters, portents and wonders there is ongoing discussion of various seventeenth-century trends discerned by historians. Is it reasonable to describe monsters as naturalized, medicalized or perhaps normalized during this period? Lorraine Daston and Katharine Park argue that by this time monsters and wonders had been explained through natural causes for centuries. Medieval researchers presented monstrous births as the result of a narrow womb, or an excess of seed, whereas natural philosophers in the late seventeenth century still sometimes read monsters as divine signs. Different modes of interpretation existed side by side, and no linear history of *disenchantment* or clear pattern of *naturalization* took monsters from an older religious framework into a newer naturalistic one or from supernatural

43 Schefferus, 'Variae historiae', chap. V. On the 'museum Schefferianum', see Burius, 'Johannes Schefferus', p. 518.

44 Löwegren, *Naturaliekabinett i Sverige*, p. 56.

45 Obsequens and Lycosthenes, *Julii Obsequentis*.

prodigies to naturalized objects. Monsters and wonders were, according to Daston and Park, rather *normalized*, related to a functional standard, and affected by a growing concern for strict regularity in nature and culture.[46]

Schefferus neither naturalized nor normalized his monsters. The prodigious boy and the monster from Lillebered were interesting, not as warnings from God or illustrations of the regularity of nature's functional standards or inviolable laws, but because in themselves they were worth seeing, remembering and knowing. Schefferus stood close to an Augustinian tradition wherein monsters, prodigies and wonders were valued for their capacity to remind people of God's presence and creative powers in the world. In 'Variae historiae' he extended what Jean Céard has called '*L'Âge d'or des prodiges*' beyond the mid-sixteenth into the late seventeenth century.[47]

Daston and Park have thoroughly examined wonders in European elite culture and discussed their value and meaning among collectors, patricians, princes, scholars, physicians and apothecaries between 1150 and 1750, but not in relation to the tradition of *exempla*, the displaying of good and bad scenarios and things for people to imitate or avoid. In this essay, I have discussed how a remarkable body or object from nature, in the same way as a spectacular history, could function as a teacher of virtue. In the early modern period things that were truly exceptional, deviating from the habits of nature, were appreciated as moral instruction for wide audiences. Schefferus celebrated the unique and peculiar things around him and associated them with knowledge and moral advancement. Instead of ignoring exceptional bodies, he willingly described them – not because they were signs of God's wrath or forewarnings of future punishments, but because they were guiding examples for people to keep in mind. He associated monsters, prodigies and wonders with intellectual processes in the beholder, just like collections of natural objects in museums or books full of spectacular histories. Strange bodies, things or phenomena in nature could influence and take root in people's minds, as images to remember, either intimidating or worth imitating. To document prodigious bodies, things and phenomena, to collect remarkable histories from the past, to contribute to a museum of wonders, and to republish ancient works on prodigies were priorities for Schefferus, who did so with accuracy and consideration.

In 'Variae historiae' we learn that rare and singular bodies, things and phenomena occasionally appear in the world and should be paid attention to. To memorize an astonishing history, object or body was to contribute to a

46 Daston and Park, *Wonders*, pp. 176, 187, 189, 202, 204-208, 214.

47 Céard, *La Nature*, p. 59.

cultural heritage and had more to do with virtue, experience and knowledge than with bad omens, prognostics and future punishments. A monster was, according to Schefferus, an extraordinary example to reflect upon – and this was far from learned definitions of such phenomena as irrelevant aberrations from a general rule. In contrast to Aristotle and the scholastics, he did not emphasize universal regularities in nature as reminders of elevated and essential truths. Instead, he encouraged contact with unique bodies, odd things and remarkable events found in history and nature.

The physicians from the Collegium Medicum may have been drawn to the fisherman's son in Norrtälje for a number of reasons but seem to have shared at least some motives with Schefferus. Instead of ignoring the body or reflecting on it in a purely theoretical sense, they observed it first-hand, drew pictures of it and examined the head, even beneath the skin. Were the investigating officials normalizing the boy, relating him to a functional standard or to some inviolable law of nature? We do not know. They might just as well have been acting in accordance with the collecting physicians, botanists, mineralogists and librarians, who cherished rare, exotic and exceptional animals, plants and minerals as paradoxical singularities of the material world. Ideally, such bodies could expand human knowledge about history, the creation, and the agency of God, man and nature.

'Variae historiae' indicates that in late-seventeenth-century Sweden, there was not a simple dichotomy between crowds gathering around ominous and frightening births and, at the other extreme, learned elites searching for universal patterns in nature and disregarding odd or irregular phenomena. Schefferus took another stance, in line with collectors of wonders, and encouraged people to let unique phenomena enter their minds. Incomparable events were approached with caution and sincere attention, and instead of dampening people's enthusiasm for monsters, Schefferus wanted to preserve their memory. As I read him, the value of the boy with a prodigious appearance lay in his capacity to bring virtue and knowledge to people, spur intellectual processes, offer guidance and improve minds. The boy in Norrtälje merited attention because he offered an education.

Works Cited

Manuscript Sources

Schefferus, Johannes, 'Variae historiae', 1670-March 1679, Uppsala University Library, MS X 292.

Primary Sources

Aelianus, Claudius, *Ailianou poikilēs historias Cl. Æliani sophistæ variæ historiæ cum notis Ioannis Schefferi* (Strasbourg, 1647).

Bromelius, Olof, *Catalogus generalis: Seu prodromus indicis specialioris ac locupletioris rerum curiosarum, tam artificialium qvam naturalium, earumq; tam exoticarum, qvam domesticarum qvæ hoc tempore inveniuntur ac servantur in pinacotheca* (Göteborg, 1698).

Columbus, Johannes (praes.), and Nicolaus Dwan (resp.), *Dissertatio academica de ominibus, quam praeside* [...] *Johanne Columbo* [...] *pro solito in philosophia titulo publico bonorum examini submittit Nicolaus Dwan Wesm. In auditorio Gustaviano ad diem Maii M.DC.LXXVI* (Stockholm, 1676).

En kort Berättelse om Den under-wärde Människian som i wår Tid uthi det Neapolitaniske Lanskapet födder och nyligen hijt till Staden ankommen är (Stockholm, 1691).

Obsequens, Julius, and Conrad Lycosthenes, *Julii Obsequentis de prodigiis liber: cum annotationibus Joannis Schefferi* [...] *accedunt Conr. Lycosthenis supplementum Obsequentis; item librorum à Scheffero editorum index* (Stockholm, 1679).

Phaedrus, 'Aesop and the Farmer', in *Fables*, by Babrius and Phaedrus, trans. Ben Edwin Perry, Loeb Classical Library 436 (Cambridge, MA: Harvard University Press, 1965), pp. 262-263.

Schefferus, Johannes, *En bok om det svenska folkets minnesvärda exempel*, introduction by Kurt Johannesson, trans. Birger Bergh (1671; Stockholm: Atlantis, 2005).

Thauvonius, Abrahamus Georgii (praes.), and Petrus Magni Gyllenius (resp.), *Disputatio physica inauguralis, de monstris* (Åbo, 1655).

Weiser, Casper Jacobsson (praes.), and Andreas Jacobi (resp.), *Disputatio physica de corporis naturalis causis per accidens, Fortuna scilicet et Casu; item de Monstris* (Lund, 1670).

Secondary Sources

Agrell, Beata, 'Att lära sig se: En didaktisk figur hos Sven Delblanc', in *Det öppna rummet: Festskrift till Merete Mazzarella den 4 februari 2005* (Helsingfors: Söderström, 2005), pp. 261-276.

Bates, A.W., *Emblematic Monsters: Unnatural Conceptions and Deformed Births in Early Modern Europe* (Amsterdam: Rodopi, 2005).

Bradley, Ritamary, 'Backgrounds of the Title Speculum in Mediaeval Literature', *Speculum* 29, no. 1 (1954), pp. 100-115.

Burius, Anders, 'Johannes Schefferus', in *Svenskt biografiskt lexikon, bd 31* (Stockholm: Svenskt biografiskt lexikon, 2002), pp. 508-520.

Céard, Jean, *La Nature et les prodiges: L'Insolite au XVIe siècle, en France* (Genève: Droz, 1977).

Dalin, A.F., *Ordbok öfver svenska språket*, 2 vols (Stockholm: A.F. Dalin, 1850-1853).

Daston, Lorraine, and Katharine Park, *Wonders and the Order of Nature, 1150-1750* (New York: Zone Books, 1998).

Ekström, Anders, *Dödens exempel: Självmordstolkningar i svenskt 1800-tal genom berättelsen om Otto Landgren* (Stockholm: Atlantis, 2000).

Findlen, Paula, *Possessing Nature: Museums, Collecting, and Scientific Culture in Early Modern Italy* (Berkeley: University of California Press, 1994).

Fredriksson, Anna, 'A Changeable World of Stone: A Glimpse into the 17th- and Early-18th-Century Discussion on the Generation of Crystals', in *Platonic Solids and Quasicrystals: Moments in the History of Crystallography*, ed. Per Cullhed (Uppsala: Uppsala universitetsbibliotek, 2013), pp. 75-85.

Häll, Mikael, *Skogsrået, näcken och djävulen: Erotiska naturväsen och demonisk sexualitet i 1600- och 1700-talens Sverige* (Stockholm: Malört, 2013).

Hellquist, Elof, *Svensk etymologisk ordbok* (Lund: Gleerup, 1922).

Hjelt, Otto E.A., *Svenska och finska medicinalverkets historia 1663-1812*, 3 vols (Helsingfors, 1891-1893).

Koselleck, Reinhart, *Futures Past: On the Semantics of Historical Time*, new ed. (New York: Columbia University Press, 2004).

Liliequist, Jonas, 'Brott, synd och straff: Tidelagsbrottet i Sverige under 1600- och 1700-talet' (PhD diss., Umeå University, 1992).

Lindroth, Sten, 'Collegium medicum och akademitanken', *Lychnos: Annual of the Swedish History of Science Society* (1943), pp. 249-253.

Löwegren, Yngve, *Naturaliekabinett i Sverige under 1700-talet: Ett bidrag till zoologiens historia* (Uppsala: Lychnos-bibliotek, 1952).

Mordhorst, Camilla, *Genstandsfortællinger: Fra Museum Wormianum til de moderne museer* (København: Museum Tusculanums Forlag, 2009).

Nationalencyklopedins ordbok, 3 vols (Höganäs: Bra böcker, 1995-1996).

Nordisk familjebok: Konversationslexikon och realencyklopedi innehållande upplysningar och förklaringar om märkvärdiga namn, föremål och begrepp, 20 vols (Stockholm, 1876-1899).

Nordisk familjebok: Konversationslexikon och realencyklopedi innehållande upplysningar och förklaringar om märkvärdiga namn, föremål och begrepp, new rev. ed., 38 vols (Stockholm: Nordisk familjeboks förl., 1904-1926).

Ordbok över svenska språket utgiven av svenska akademien, 38 vols (Lund: Gleerupska univ.- bokh., 1893-).

Pomian, Krzysztof, *Collectors and Curiosities: Paris and Venice, 1500-1800*, trans. Elizabeth Wiles-Portier (Cambridge: Polity Press, 1990).

Savin, Kristiina, 'Anekdoter om dygd: Värdenas retorik i Johannes Schefferus bok om det svenska folkets minnesvärda exempel (1671)', in *Förmoderna livshållningar: Dygder, värden och kunskapsvägar från antiken till upplysningen*, ed. M. Lindstedt Cronberg and C. Stenqvist (Lund: Nordic Academic Press, 2008), pp. 234-258.
Secord, James A., 'Knowledge in Transit', *Isis* 95, no. 4 (2004), pp. 654-672.

About the Author

Maja Bondestam is Associate Professor in History of Science and Ideas at Uppsala University. She has published books and articles on themes including politics of the maturing body, the history of the Swedish hermaphrodite, botanical classification, the language of Carl Linnaeus and gendered norms in medical advice literature.

7. Ambiguous and Transitional Bodies: Stillbirth in Stockholm, 1691-1724[1]

Tove Paulsson Holmberg

Abstract
This essay explores the connection between discourses and images of unborn corporeality and early modern perinatal loss. Stressing the ambiguous and conditional status of unborn infants in birth manuals published by Swedish physician and man-midwife Johan von Hoorn (1662-1724), it analyses medical and religious emergency practices related to stillbirth: decoding signs of decay and viability, podalic version, resuscitation techniques, obstetric surgery and emergency baptism. The results suggest that discourses and images of obstructed and stillborn infants were influenced by the determination to intervene manually and conjured up by haptic experiences conditioned by specific limitations and possibilities that characterized birth practices in this context.

Keywords: perinatal mortality, seventeenth-century Sweden, Johan von Hoorn, birth manuals, obstetric intervention, emergency baptism

But grant that the child come into the world of it selfe, without the help either of chirurgion or Midwife: yet (as it is commonly said,) he drawes his death after him: the which may bee plainly perceived by the cries and laments which he maketh as soone as hee seeth the light, as if hee craved for help and succour.
– Jacques Guillemeau, *Child-Birth*, 1635

From this we can learn: First, how uncertain it is to judge a child dead, which does not move, since it sometimes can be so pressed together by the labour pains that it cannot move its limbs, and yet live.
– Johan von Hoorn, *The Twenne Gudfruchtige* [...] *SIPHRA och PUA*, 1719

1 This work was supported by Helge Ax:son Johnson Foundation. All translations are by the author, unless stated otherwise.

Bondestam, M. (ed.), *Exceptional Bodies in Early Modern Culture: Concepts of Monstrosity before the Advent of the Normal*. Taylor & Francis Group, 2020
DOI 10.5117/9789463721745_CH07

Birth is a dangerous and dynamic event resulting in new life, as well as in death and loss. As distinct as the birth transition may seem, it remains essentially a process. The term 'perinatal' defines the phase beginning in late pregnancy when the fetus has potential to survive the delivery, and ending, roughly, seven days after birth, demarcating the period when the child gradually emerges and stabilizes itself in the world of the living.

This chapter explores the exceptional and strange bodies of early modern perinatal children from the perspective of liminality and loss. Fetal and infant growth and separation are precarious processes composed of many stages, turning points and transformations. If premodern monstrosity, as argued by Michel Foucault, was defined by transgressive and transboundary qualities, fetal and infant concepts and imagery from this era to some degree placed perinatal bodies in the monstrous realm.[2] They represented an existence waiting to emerge and consolidate, or dissolve and move on. Early modern European birth practices were conditioned by the fundamental uncertainty of the signs of viability and decay emanating from fetal and infant bodies absorbed in processes of fulfilment and separation, blurring the line between life and death. The aim of this chapter is to make concepts of viability part of studies on monstrous and exceptional bodies and practices and to trace the presence of death, decay and transformation in discourses and images of the early modern Swedish perinatal child.

Early modern unborn entities were essentially strange, growing and residing in concealment: at the borders of life.[3] Their fragile and unstable corporeality 'echoed the macrocosmic order' of the perilous human condition. From the moment they manifested life by 'quickening', their liminal condition was monitored and their successful separation from the maternal body was anxiously pursued. The anticipated new life was embraced in terms of abundance, vigour and potentiality. Yet unborn corporeality was deeply tainted by the dark prospect of abortive and nonviable ends. And however inevitably they might be lost, the management of wasted and dying fetuses and infants was influenced by urgent interventions to safeguard the salvation of their souls. Negotiating the status of the unborn, birth practitioners pursued survival in both the physical and the eternal dimension. Detailed observations of the ambiguous signs emanating from

2 Foucault, *Abnormal*, pp. 63-64.

3 In her seminal work *Purity and Danger: An Analysis of Concepts of Pollution and Taboo*, the anthropologist Mary Douglas underlines the cross-cultural status of the unborn as marginal creatures, 'both vulnerable and dangerous'. Douglas, *Purity and Danger*, p. 95.

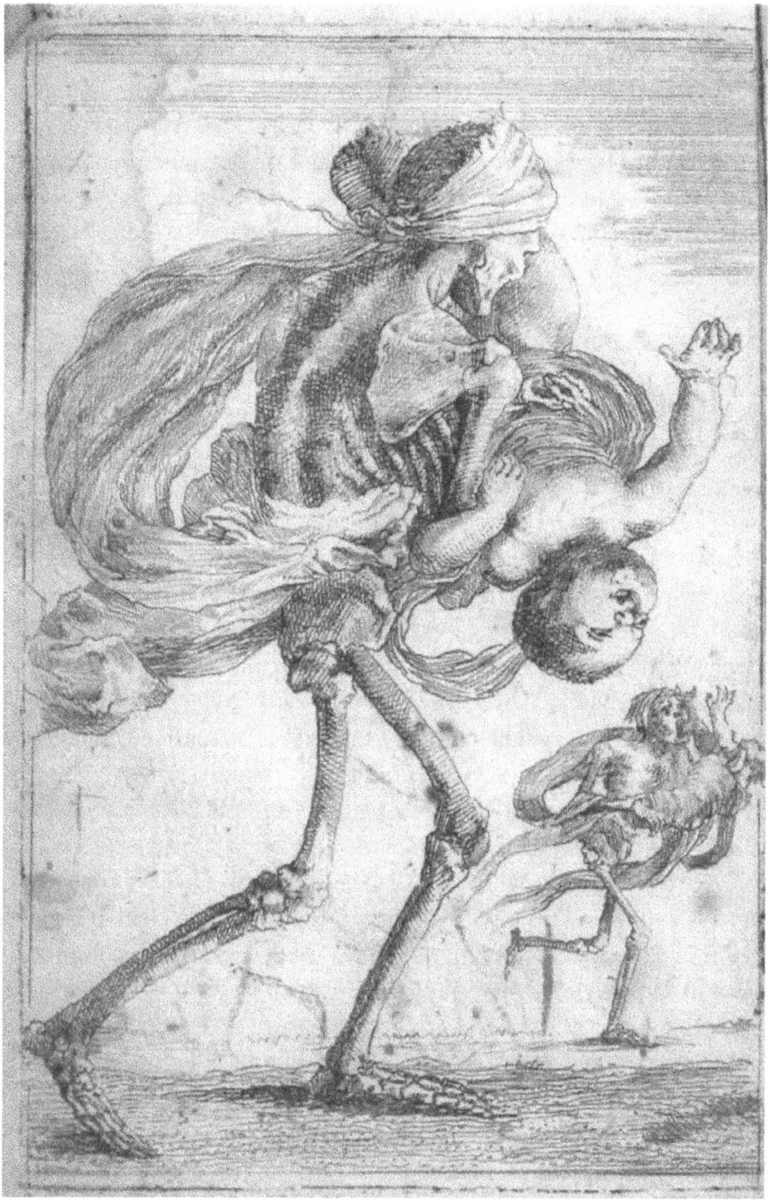

Figure 7.1. Death and the infant: The child has a dull expression in its chubby face. Death squeezes it hard to her emaciated breast. She turns her back at us and increases her speed. Physician Lars Roberg, who inserted her portrait in Lijkrevningstavlor (1719), knew her well. "Myself beeing the eldest, I lost two Brothers in their first childhood, and three Sisters", he commented in his memoirs.[4] Frontispiece, Lars Roberg, *Profess. d:r Laur. Roberg's Lijkrevnings tavlor [...]* (Stockholm, 1718). Photograph: Helena Backman.

4 Quoted from Åke Dintler, *Lars Roberg: Akademiska sjukhusets grundare* (Uppsala, 1959), p. 16.

living and dead perinatal bodies were central to this endeavour. In the following, close reading of birth manuals published by the Swedish man-midwife, physician and teacher of midwives Johan von Hoorn (1662-1724) will be used to explore how discourses and practices related to late fetal and intrapartum mortality reveal the interaction between medical and religious expectations, hopes and limitations concerning physical and spiritual survival in late-seventeenth- and early-eighteenth-century Sweden.

Birth manuals, perinatal mortality and obstetric intervention

The extent of perinatal loss in early modern contexts is hard to assess, because of the imprecise categories used and the silence and fragmentation of the sources.[5] Yet this particular type of mortality has been acknowledged as having a fundamental bearing upon early modern worldviews.[6] Analysing the management of childbirth, scholars in cultural and medical history have observed how the dangers of reproduction shaped early modern European fetal and infant concepts and imagery.[7] This chapter focuses on death related to the birth transition, that is, *stillbirth*. Highlighting the final separation of the maternal body and the supposedly viable, fully developed child, it traces the prospect of nurturing and giving birth to the lifeless and the dead, rather than to the deviant, unique, and thought-provoking bodies described by Bondestam in chapter six in this volume.[8] The monstrosity at focus here is the double presence of life and death in perinatal bodies, which was exceptional and remarkable in itself, but also deeply problematic to the performance of religious transition rites. Since survival of mother and child in a complicated birth depended on decoding signs of unborn vitality and decay before, during and after birth, descriptions of such signs and adequate interventions were a central feature of obstetric textbooks and manuals, the publication of which grew substantially in seventeenth-century Europe.

Early modern birth manuals were a diversified genre of publication devoted to the theory and practice of birth, targeting both practitioners and the public. Though such publications remain biased and self-promoting, they have been widely used by historians to analyse various aspects of early

5 Woods, *Death before Birth*.

6 Imhof, *Lost Worlds*; Gélis, *Les enfants*.

7 For example, Duden, *The Woman*; Gélis, *History of Childbirth*.

8 See Bondestam, 'An Education', in this volume.

modern reproduction and obstetrics.[9] Here, observations of, and practices related to, fetal vitality and decay will be used to illuminate the ambiguous and fluid corporeality of perinatal children in Stockholm in the decades around 1700.

The author discussed below, Johan von Hoorn, left Stockholm as a teenager in 1679 and spent twelve years in Leiden, Amsterdam, and Paris, completing his training in medicine, surgery and midwifery. In 1690 he defended his thesis, *De partu praeternaturali*, at Leiden University. After returning to Sweden in 1691, he spent three decades practising medicine in Stockholm. During these years Von Hoorn worked steadily to transform Swedish midwifery through private and public training of individual midwives, finally managing to establish a set of official regulations for the profession in 1711. He was the author of three birth manuals in five editions in the vernacular,[10] all promoting an interventionist obstetrics based on anatomical knowledge, internal examination of pregnant and parturient women, and techniques of manipulating and turning children in abnormal fetal presentations (i.e. podalic version).[11]

The birth manuals of Von Hoorn conform to the variations and particulars of the genre in the decades around 1700. In style and content, they correspond with contemporary European authors, mainly the French accoucheurs François Mauriceau and Paul Portal, the German midwife Justine Siegemund and the Dutch surgeon and orthopaedist Hendrik van Deventer. Three publications include proper case studies: the second (1719) and third (1726) editions of *SIPHRA och PUA* (13 cases in the second edition, and 30 in the third) and *Then Swenska Wälöfwade Jorde-Gummans Andra Deel* (1723), a translation of Portal's *La Pratique des accouchemens* (1680), describing 80 Parisian cases with commentary by Von Hoorn that frequently makes references to similar cases experienced by the translator himself.

All case studies deal with labour dystocia, difficult and complicated birth. They concern the serious ethical and technical problem of the so-called obstetrical dilemma, and fetal and intrapartum death permeates them through and through.

9 Marland, *Mother and Child*; Wilson, *The Making*; Keller, 'The Subject of Touch'; McTavish, *Childbirth*; Woods, *Death before Birth*; Churchill, *Female Patients*.

10 Von Hoorn, *Den Swenska Wäl-öfwade Jord-Gumman* (1697); Von Hoorn, *The Twenne Gudfruchtige* [...] *SIPHRA och PUA* (1715); Von Hoorn, *The Twenne Gudfruchtige* [...] *SIPHRA och PUA* (1719); Von Hoorn, *Then Swenska Wälöfwade Jorde-Gummans Andra Deel* (1723); Von Hoorn, *Die Zwo um ihrer Gottesfurcht* [...] *Siphra und Pua* (1726).

11 Djurberg, *Läkaren Johan von Hoorn*; Paulsson Holmberg, *Onaturlig födelse*.

Obstetric anxiety and reality

The obstetrical dilemma illustrates the evolutionary negotiation between the size of the unborn head and the width of the maternal pelvis that makes human reproduction to some degree inherently dangerous. Observing the high risk in humans in contrast to the rest of the natural world, so-called traditional societies have often favoured metaphysical and religious explanations.[12] In early modern Europe all deaths related to the birth transition were explained as part of the human condition after the Fall. Painful and dangerous delivery was ordained by God as a punishment for original sin, and the suffering and death of individual mothers and children were in most part accepted as unavoidable. However, stoic endurance in the face of loss and bereavement does not rule out resolution and the will to fight. Manifestations of 'obstetric anxiety' surface in various contexts in seventeenth-century European culture.[13] These manifestations indicate that the dangers of childbirth, for various reasons, were increasingly viewed as disturbing the equilibrium.

Labour dystocia is a complex phenomenon that depends on a combination of physiological and cultural factors. Though many initially slow and extended deliveries end with the mother giving birth naturally, some complications require intervention if both mother and child are to survive unharmed. In early modern terminology, difficult and obstructed deliveries, where the forces of nature had failed and art – manual and surgical intervention – was deemed necessary, were labelled 'unnatural'.

Seventeenth-century nature was a manifestation of God, the best possible order, wise and good, pervaded by customs but occasionally open for modifications and exceptions. In a universe full of aims and meanings, deviances from expected patterns, such as 'unnatural' birth, evoked curiosity and intellectual interest. A growing volume of medical publications on the dynamic separation process of mother and child emerged, pursuing observation, recording, analysis, and, in particular, intervention.

In the late seventeenth century, the use of interventionist techniques and manipulations became more common, due to the rise of male practitioners, mainly surgeons, making 'unnatural delivery' their main occupation, as well as the trend towards professionalization for urban midwives. The increased use of interventionist methods was influenced by a new understanding of the pelvis and its effects on labour dystocia. After anatomists finally

12 Bates and Turner, 'Imagery and Symbolism', p. 91.

13 Schwartz, *Milton*, chap. 2.

disproved the ancient notion that the pelvic joints open to aid the passage of the child, the problem of obstructed birth was reinvented.[14] The pelvis emerged as a deciding factor, and it was recognized that some women were, for mechanical reasons, incapable of giving birth naturally. The survival of mother and child in such cases now became the responsibility of the birth practitioner.

This chapter reflects concepts and images of perinatal corporeality influenced by the specific conditions that governed discourses and practices of birth from around 1650, when interventionist techniques developed in tandem with the professional identities of birth practitioners, to the 1730s, when midwifery forceps were introduced. It was an art characterized by limitations. Instruments that could extract the child unharmed were non-existent. In desperate cases, separation could only be effected by sacrificing either mother or child. Expectations of suffering and loss were part of the fabric of existence, a necessary coping strategy against despair. With this in mind we return to the obstructed unborn and Von Hoorn's manuals. How did the birth practitioner describe this creature and its survival prospects?

The spectre of death

That a fetus can die in the womb of the mother is confirmed by everyday experience.
– Johan von Hoorn, *Den Swenska Wäl-öfwade Jord-Gumman*, 1697

Descriptions of stillborn infants often use metaphors that stress liminality, alienation, poise and serenity. The stillborn is a promise unfulfilled: a familiar stranger, hesitating for a moment, only to turn back and disappear in the darkness. It is a glimpse of a restful face forever lost in the sleep of death. This is the image of an innocent and dignified creature of another world, having the aura of a recently deceased person, in whom the appearance of life still lingers on.

Late-seventeenth-century obstetric emergencies sometimes resulted in the birth of such a child. But they also produced mutilated bodies with broken skulls, swollen bodies, bodies with blackened or whitened limbs, decomposing and rotten bodies falling apart in the hands of practitioners like 'cooked meat'. Stillborn children could thus be either long dead and corrupted, recently deceased, or something in between. Fetal death is generally linked to genetic defects or poor maternal health, while intrapartum

14 Eccles, *Obstetrics and Gynaecology*, p. 105.

and neonatal mortality depend on the trauma of birth.[15] In early modern contexts, some losses in the latter category were preventable, while others were directly connected to the interventionist birth practices used, a fact that did not escape the affected parties.

The central argument used by Von Hoorn and other promoters of manual and surgical intervention in the last decades of the seventeenth century was that it saved the life of the mother and lessened her injuries. Interventionist practices and techniques could be described as necessary instruments and acts directed towards dead fetuses threatening to kill their suffering mothers. By starting from the premise that surgical instruments by definition are used on dead children, the critique against them was disarmed, and the fundamental uncertainty of the dangerous predicament of the unborn child remained hidden.

There is a dark, melancholy sense of danger and premonition of loss in the birth manuals of Von Hoorn, colouring statements about the perinatal child, emphasizing its threatened, conditional character. In the thesis (*De partu praeternaturali* [1690]), the child was characterized by dark metaphors and associations: it has 'one foot on Charon's ferry', is 'liberated from the jaws of death', 'revoked and revived from the misery', or 'withdrawn from Orcus'. When the author on a single occasion describes how an infant surprises everyone by screaming, and calls the sound 'more wonderful than the most beautiful music', his choice of words merely emphasizes the echoing absence of images that underline infant strength and vitality in other parts of the text.[16]

In his early years of practicing midwifery, Von Hoorn focused on promoting early intervention, thus supposedly preventing the extreme consequences of obstruction and neglect. The self-presentation and selection of focus in the later manuals suggests, however, that his practice increasingly became oriented towards hopeless and desperate cases. Since this meant performing intrauterine surgery, the examination and analysis of the unborn head, face, limbs, and umbilical cord gradually became paramount. In *Den Swenska Wäl-öfwade Jord-Gumman* (1697), Von Hoorn stated that signs of fetal death are more reliable than signs of intrapartum death, and that deciphering the latter often leads to 'disagreement and quarrel' among those present. A child deeply descended and fixed in the pelvis may be unable to move, and thus be declared dead, even though it can survive for days in this position. Such a fetus challenged not only the distinction between mother and child

15 Woods, *Death before Birth*, p. 5.
16 Von Hoorn, *De partu praeternaturali*, p. [38].

but also that between life and death. ‘Many lamentable examples’ have revealed how difficult it is to interpret its status. But if the midwife feels no movement in the tongue, nor pulsation in fontanelle, neck, arm, leg or umbilical cord, the child is ‘unerringly dead’.[17] She may then proceed with ‘audacity’, concentrating on delivering the mother with as little pain as possible, not having to show any ‘tenderness’ towards the dead child.[18] In obstructed birth by the head, however, none of the body parts mentioned above are available for examination. The author thus hesitates and ends with a warning – it is ‘better and more secure’ to treat a dead child as living, than to risk that one might ‘butcher’ a living child.[19]

Recognizing signs of fetal death was crucial, since no one opposed methods that liberated the mother from the remains of a dead child. The reason that separation in abnormal fetal presentations generally was successful was the accessibility of unborn limbs. Von Hoorn’s case studies abound with arm, foot, and umbilical cord presentations which result in survival and complete recovery of the mother, since distinct signs of decay in protruding infant body parts enabled instant intervention.

Obstructed birth by the head, by contrast, was invariably linked to hesitation and delay. Assessing various methods of examination in *SIPHRA och PUA* (1715), Von Hoorn rejected most signs of fetal death in this complication as ‘of no value, since they are no more than unsure surmises’. The only sign he approved of was a green and odorous substance appearing on cloths pressed against the vagina.[20] But given that the substance was most likely secreted from a child that had been some time dead, he cautioned against waiting for this sign to appear. Instead, he made a bold statement: in desperate cases midwives may treat the unborn as dead, destroy the head with a pair of scissors, and extract the body by means of this handle.[21] This last resort of birth practitioners was included in the official regulations for midwives from 1711.[22] Giving licensed midwives the right to use sharp instruments violated the ancient boundary between surgeon and midwife that many contemporary practitioners tried to uphold and testifies to the perceived need of an experienced birth practitioner to support intervention in desperate emergency cases. It was a position that stated that leaving the mother undelivered was unacceptable. In such a context, recognizing vital signs

17 Von Hoorn, *Den Swenska Wäl-öfwade Jord-Gumman* (1697), p. 53.
18 Ibid., p. 57.
19 Ibid., p. 59f.
20 Von Hoorn, *The Twenne Gudfruchtige* [...] *SIPHRA och PUA* (1715), p. 19.
21 Ibid., p. 109f.
22 *Reglemente och Förordning*, p. 10.

in unborn bodies clearly emerged as a crucial ability of birth practitioners, enabling prompt intervention, as illustrated below in the observations describing obstetric emergency practices in Stockholm and Paris.

Intervention in Stockholm and Paris

> *When I remember the wife earlier alluded to, who was so pitifully neglected for the uncertain life of her child, and who begged with such heart-moving prayers and touching gestures, until she lost her mind, that someone would deliver her, and that it must be better to save one life (in her own words) than to lose both; so can I admit: that my entire body shivers, [on the recollection] that I was not allowed to deliver her, when I requested it, and save her life, as I have later done with many other persons.*
> – Johan von Hoorn, *Then Swenska Wälöfwade Jorde-Gummans Andra Deel*, 1723

Performing the separation of maternal and fetal bodies in obstructed birth remained conditioned by several factors. Von Hoorn narrated these factors, as well as the processes of examination and intervention, in the format of case studies. The 80 cases from Paris (1723) and 30 cases from Stockholm (1726) represented recurring problems carefully selected and edited by the author, who states that they 'mirror the entire content of the art'.[23] They allow a general overview of methods and techniques related to emergency practices: the incidence of early and late intervention and the outcomes and causes of death observed.[24]

Then Swenska Wälöfwade Jorde-Gummans Andra Deel (1723) consists of 80 observations by surgeon Paul Portal in 1660s Paris, recording 74 deliveries (included eight cases of twins and two cases of triplets), describing the birth of 86 children. In thirteen cases explicit information on the outcome for the child ('was dead', 'was living', 'was baptized in church') is lacking. Eliminating these observations, 73 cases remain, of which 35 children survived birth. In four cases, the newborn was deadly weakened and perished soon ('after half an hour', 'briefly after baptism'). One child was resuscitated by Portal 'after lying without any movement or pulsation of the heart and the cord for more than a quarter of an hour'. The number of stillborn was 38; of which thirteen were rotten, three 'deformed', six premature (of which three cases connected to placenta previa). In two cases of multiple birth, at least one child was dead and 'unripe'. Only four cases of infant death resulted from

23 Von Hoorn, *Then Swenska Wälöfwade Jorde-Gummans Andra Deel* (1723), p. 5.
24 Paulsson Holmberg, *Onaturlig födelse*, p. 224.

mistakes committed by birth practitioners. Of these, two children died in relation to podalic version, and one twin bled to death with its mother, since the midwife did not expect a second child. And in a particularly grim case, Portal witnessed a mother die after a fellow surgeon had dismembered her unborn child in utero and left her fatally wounded.

The principal cause of complicated birth in the Parisian cases was abnormal fetal presentations (54 per cent) followed by haemorrhage (19 per cent). The remaining cases dealt with fits, symptoms of fetal decay and obstructed birth by the head. In eight cases (11 per cent) instruments were used to extract the child: two cases of obstructed birth by the head (case no. 17, no. 25), one failed version (no. 21), two deformed and dead children (no. 30, no. 32), two rotten children (no. 57, no. 75) and one failed attempt to operate on an unborn child, performed by an unnamed surgeon (no. 63). The observations stress the merits of podalic version, which was tried in two-thirds of all cases, resulting in the successful delivery of almost all children, dead or alive, and survival of the mother.

In Portal's observations nearly half of the interventions resulted in a living child. The selected cases from Stockholm have a much darker character. Of 29 deliveries, only five children were born alive. Three of the survivors were extremely weak and were resuscitated, by the author himself or by attending midwives.

All the remaining cases resulted in a stillbirth. Twelve children were judged dead by the practitioner on his arrival (of which three were distinctly rotten and six had died in prolonged labour after mistakes committed by birth practitioners); three were judged alive but emerged dead; five were impossible to examine; two were distinctly alive at the onset of labour, but succumbed in the birth passage. In two cases, Von Hoorn mutilated children of uncertain status to save the life of the mother.

When Von Hoorn speculates on causes of death, narrow pelvises, stiff and hard genital parts and pressure against the umbilical cord emerge as principal explanations. But prolonged labour in itself could also kill the child by exercising compression, as could the violence used to perform version.

In ten cases instruments were used to separate mother and child. Of these, only three children were 'uncertain'. An unborn infant with a deformed leg was extracted with a hook cautiously placed in the thigh: 'Since I thought: Does the child live, so can it not die because of this; and as soon as it is born I will dab the thigh with warm brandy.'[25] In all the remaining cases, labour had been very extended, which gave reason to believe that

25 Von Hoorn, *Die Zwo um ihrer Gottesfurcht* [...] *Siphra und Pua* (1726), p. 214.

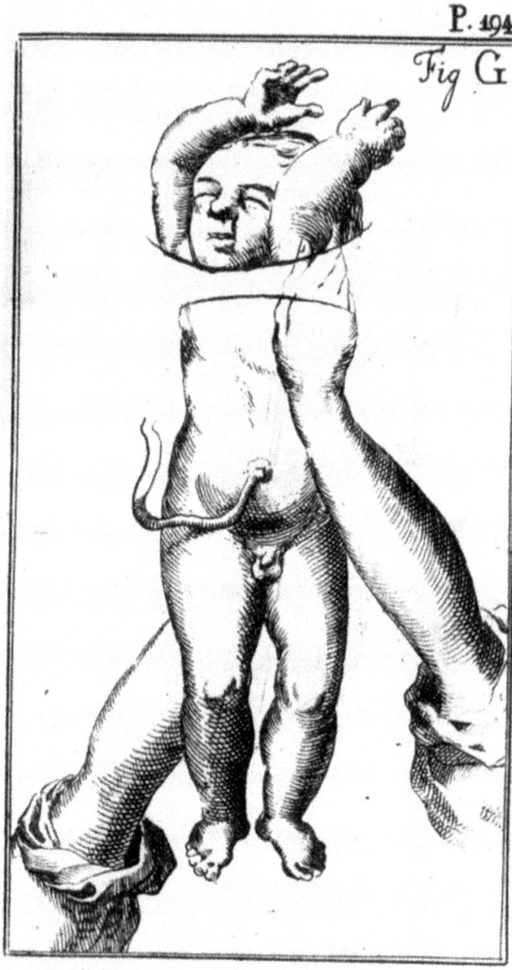

Figure 7.2. Podalic version demands great mental and physical strength of the performer. He or she who wants to try it must "not stand sleeping, and have the vigor, and the heart, to carry it through".[27] Johan von Hoorn, *Den Swenska Wäl-öfwade Jord-Gumman [...]* (Stockholm, 1697). Photograph: Lund University Library (LUB).

the child was wasted. A large, deeply wedged child presenting a shoulder was decapitated and quartered. And in the final observation describing a case of obstructed birth by the head, where Von Hoorn extracted the child with an instrument placed in the broken skull, he closed with a warning: 'in unnecessary cases, do not hasten to the final, and for the child, lethal method, but move *gradatim*, or step-by-step, from the mild to the severe'.[26]

26 Von Hoorn, *The Twenne Gudfruchtige* [...] *SIPHRA och PUA* (1715), p. 109f.

27 Von Hoorn 1697, p. 220.

Judging from these obstetric narratives, many unborn children handled by birth practitioners were already dead, and yet more died during labour, often from causes that were difficult to prevent. Mothers with deformed bodies ('narrow pelvises') often gave birth to dead children. When large children were wedged in the birth passage by violent labour pains, they often died of asphyxia due to pressure against the umbilical cord, and haemorrhage caused by placenta previa almost always resulted in a stillbirth. But the observations also reveal that early manual intervention in abnormal presentations, that is, podalic version, was generally successful, and often resulted in the survival of both mother and child.

Unfortunately, podalic version was a difficult technique to master. If performed after the water had broken, it could be impossible to force the child back. Turning the child in arm presentations sometimes required that birth practitioners 'removed' the arm to be able to reach the feet. And once turned, the unborn head could be separated from the body and remain in the uterus, particularly if the child came out twisted.

In arm presentations, the difference between the swollen 'plump' limb of a living child and the pale, consumed limb of the dead determined the methods used (or avoided) by the author. With the possible exception of rotten and corrupted fetuses, Von Hoorn always struggled to deliver the child intact: 'It seems so cruel and shocking to assault and butcher a child, and you terrify them [the mothers] from the helpful hands of men,' he pondered in the introduction to his translation of Portal.[28] The butchered unborn infant was a picture of total loss, void of consolation. It is significant that narrations of interventions where dismemberment takes place are fragmentary and incomplete. Commenting upon the subject of obstetric surgery in 1708, Von Hoorn stated that 'it is [perhaps] better to emulate the skilful poets who direct the eyes of the public away from that which is distasteful to behold'.[29] Possibly he hesitated to describe critical surgical techniques in print, especially in the manuals that openly addressed an audience of midwives. Merely alluding to this surgical competence may have been a way to inform readers – some of them probably being students of surgery – that the author possessed this dangerous knowledge, and might perform the techniques or teach them to a select audience of students and apprentices.[30]

The unstated implication of the obstetric emergency narratives, though, recurrently reminded readers of the indistinct signs of fetal life. Explicit signs

28 Von Hoorn, *Then Swenska Wälöfwade Jorde-Gummans Andra Deel* (1723), p. [13].
29 Von Hoorn, *Anatomes publicae*, p. [95].
30 Paulsson Holmberg, *Onaturlig födelse*, p. 138f.

of fetal decay were always described in the case studies, and in dubious cases, the process of assessment and the outcome were meticulously recorded. The ability to decode signs of fetal and infant decay was important to another medical-legal context that Von Hoorn participated in: investigations of suspected infanticide. In 1718, he described himself as a person who during 30 years of practice had handled 'several living, half-dead, and dead children', and as city physician had examined 'many illegitimate dead-born children'.[31] As for the latter, determining causes of death could be very hard, since the remains had often been severely broken down. To underline this point, Von Hoorn reinforced his argument with observations from his childbirth practice. His underlying assumption in these reflections is that breathing is a vital requirement. Von Hoorn suggests that intrapartum death often results from intrauterine obstruction of the umbilical cord. To subsequently prove that such blockage has taken place is described as impossible. Another problem addressed is how to distinguish between the actual stillborn and children who only 'seem dead'. Podalic version may leave infants so weakened that

> they do not breathe, and no movement in the cord or veins can be perceived, so that you must judge them completely dead, but they live anyway. I have often seen such children so weak, that I have held it impossible that anyone might be able to revive them, yet the midwife, with her persevering and indefatigable nursing, has evoked life in them again.[32]

The flickering, faint light of the newborn, managed and guarded by the midwife for the purpose that overshadowed all others: enabling baptism.

Temporary survival and salvation

> *As she helps them enter the world alive, she promotes them to the holy baptism, so that these little ones, that are conceived in sin, may be washed clean in the precious blood of the Saviour. Which is such a great act of benefaction, that it is not possible to describe it with the pen.*
>
> – Johan von Hoorn, *Den Swenska Wäl-öfwade Jord-Gumman*, 1697

Some children hesitated on the threshold of life. Others struggled so hard to force the transition that they seemed quite dead, 'but yet [are] living'.

31 Von Hoorn, *Bref til* [...] *Anatomiæ Professorn Herr Magnus Bromell*, p. 2.
32 Ibid., p. 13.

Observing faint signs of life in these liminal creatures had been the duty of the midwife since time immemorial. If there was any hope, she had to perform emergency baptism and secure the child a place in the safe afterlife of eternity.

The central sacrament of baptism was an enduring dilemma in early modern Europe. In guarding the dignity of the most essential of Christian rites, the church had to defend the uncertain fate of all individuals deprived of it. Emerging from this necessary demarcation was the conclusion that the stillborn could not receive salvation. Instead of reuniting with their families in the afterlife, they went to a particular place called the 'children's Limbo'. To meet the demands of desperate parents midwives performed emergency baptism in utero and baptized long-dead children who displayed supposed 'life signs'.[33] In Lutheran countries like Sweden, baptismal doctrine demanded that children be 'completely born' and display distinct signs of life to receive the sacrament. Moreover, protestant theologians concluded that the fate of stillborn children, as well as all dead persons, must remain 'unknown'. Anxious parents were reassured that if they commended their unborn to the hands of God, he would most likely accept them anyway: 'For He does not look so much upon external deeds, which can by many means often be hindered, but upon the will and the heart.'[34] The pressure to perform emergency baptism in dubious cases thus lessened, and the practice of stabilizing weak children first became more prominent.[35] And given that interventionist birth practices often left practitioners with lifeless and weakened newborns, practices of intervention, emergency baptism and resuscitation developed in tandem.

That podalic version resulted in an increased need for reanimation is evident from the early manuals of Von Hoorn, which devote entire chapters to the subject. Delivering the child feet first may be hazardous. If the head gets stuck, amniotic fluid can enter the lungs. Podalic version also increases the risk of pressure against the umbilical cord, with resulting asphyxia. Von Hoorn makes it clear that the midwife must prepare herself for hard work if she wants to save the child. It is in her mind before she starts her manipulations: 'And she knows already: that the child is commonly weak' or she 'fears that it may be deadly weak, and as if altogether extinguished'.[36] The chapter 'How to Revive a New-Born Child' (1697) reveals the interplay between available

33 Gélis, *Les enfants*.

34 *Laurentius Petris Kyrkoordning av år 1571*, p. 59.

35 Grell, 'The Protestant Imperative', p. 53; Cressy, *Birth*, p. 123.

36 Von Hoorn, *The Twenne Gudfruchtige* [...] *SIPHRA och PUA* (1715), p. 104.

techniques of resuscitation, life signs and emergency baptism. The author initially observes that slow and obstructed delivery often results in weak and lifeless children. To escape censure the midwife must state this to the attendant family. She then prepares herself with a bowl of clean water, a brush, an onion, a bottle of wine, and various substances and pharmaceuticals. After the separation, she takes the infant in her lap and examines it closely. If there seems to be hope of life, she clears mouth and throat to aid breathing. If she then notices stronger vital signs, she immediately proceeds to baptize the child. But if there is doubt, she must use all her powers to revive the child further by irritating its face with the substances and stimulating the soles of its feet with the brush. When she finally observes 'more life', she may baptize the child. This decision must be approved of by other persons present: 'So that she can be free from censure, as if she had abused the holy [sacrament of] baptism, and baptized a dead child.'[37]

Stillborn infants lacking vital signs may still have received emergency baptism, provided that they were not evidently dead. Mutilated fetal bodies, though, could never be accepted as 'potentially alive'. The case studies reveal, as argued before, the distinct risk of mutilating the unborn in unnatural delivery: in particular in arm presentations, where the protruding limb had to be removed; failed versions, where the trunk of the body had to be quartered, and obstructed birth by the head, where the skull of the child had to be destroyed to perform separation. Given the violence used in connection with these manipulations and techniques, it is reasonable to suggest that an important merit of forceps was their ability to deliver dead children intact, thus sparing all present the frightening view of butchered infant body parts, which affected the reputation of the obstetric surgeon so badly.

Still, the tolerated 'necessary violence' of surgeons may explain the complete absence of religious representatives and incidents of emergency baptism in the case studies, as well as the fact that remarkably few children were revived, despite the knowledge of the dubious character of signs of vitality and decay. Presumably, they were clearly and indisputably dead after being subjected to the violent assaults of desperate birth practitioners.

In his commentary to Portal's 25th observation, Von Hoorn uses the term *feg* to characterize children that are stuck and deeply wedged in the birth passage. The child is doomed and lost, 'predetermined for death'. The surgeon who attacks its body only hastens its 'timely' death.

This announcement reveals that saving the mother is non-negotiable to the author. If practitioners do not want to abandon her in this vulnerable

37 Von Hoorn, *Den Swenska Wäl-öfwade Jord-Gumman* (1697), p. 271f.

situation and leave her dying with the child inside her, then they must be prepared to 'harm and wound the child to death', he forcefully insists. The alternative – to remove the child with Caesarean section – is not mentioned. This means in reality a defence for therapeutic abortion.

The tension of the texts becomes visible in the balance. What is possible; what is reasonable; what is unacceptable. Before separation, the priority is the mother; after separation, the child. This child, who by surviving the passage and entering the world as an individual and the living image of God, has inviolable rights, 'the blood of whom; after worldly and divine law, cannot be spilled without revenge'.[38]

Birth thus appears as a distinct boundary, a before and an after, a marked line. Before the child has been separated from the mother and breathes by itself, it must cede preference to her. Breathing is, according to the doctor, a '*requisitum essentiale*' for life. A person sacrificing the child in a desperate obstetric emergency, in hopes of saving the life of the mother, could therefore not be defined as a murderer, but rather as someone 'who has stolen gold from a person, who would, in time, inherit gold; but yet does not own it'.[39]

The intervening practitioner was operating in the realm of 'unnatural' procedures. And while death and loss in obstructed and complicated birth remained part of the natural order, a complete separation and temporary live birth preserved the moral order by securing baptism, and spiritual survival, of the child. Here the exceptional state of perinatal bodies discloses their monstrous qualities, which, according to Foucault, demands not only transgressions of natural limits and classifications, but also the disturbing of civil and religious interdictions.[40] It is, however, in the quote above, not the perinatal child who is violating the moral order but the obstetrician. When he sacrificed the child, he had stolen gold and performed in a *juridical-natural* activity, troubling both natural boundaries and religious claims.

Arguing in defence of intervention, Von Hoorn uses quotes from Mauriceau, Tertullian and Deventer to support his view that, in certain cases, 'shortening' of the insecure child's life 'with good conscience can and should be executed to save the life of the mother'.[41]

Yet he hesitates, as if fearing his own conclusions. Can surgical intervention that kills the unborn ever be combined with a 'good conscience'? In order to justify his recommendations, Von Hoorn claims that he has consulted

38 Von Hoorn, *Then Swenska Wälöfwade Jorde-Gummans Andra Deel* (1723), p. 73.
39 Ibid.
40 Foucault, *Abnormal*, pp. 63-64.
41 Von Hoorn, *Then Swenska Wälöfwade Jorde-Gummans Andra Deel* (1723), p. 75.

'theologians and teachers of the word of God, as men of conscience, about their meaning', from whom he supposedly received the pragmatic answer that 'all reasonable persons' facing this difficult dilemma must try to save the only life they are able to save – that of the mother.[42]

In developing his argument supporting the rights of 'lawfully appointed accoucheurs' to terminate the life of the child in such emergency situations, Von Hoorn uses parables that put his image of the conditional, already lost child in sharp relief. The unborn is reduced to 'a limb, or part of the woman' and is compared to gynaecological tumours such as 'mola uterina, mamma cancrosa, scirrus cancrosus [...] who all owe their maintenance and life to the woman; but nonetheless must be removed'. From a medical perspective, this entity, which does not breathe by itself and receives nourishment from a 'foster mother', cannot be regarded as a 'real human being'. In case that the unborn infant is attributed human status, there are two options. Either 'such a child who [...] is the enemy of the woman, and threatens her life' may be treated as a potential 'mother slayer', and in that case, it is the duty of birth practitioners to execute the death sentence. Or the child could be held '*absolute* for a dead fetus'; it is a sensible solution that reduces the risk of losing the mother. Finally, Von Hoorn emphasizes that it is the official duty of physicians 'to remove all harmful, which can drag man to his grave'.[43]

To hesitate is to hope that miracles happen. It means defending the right of the liminal child to 'receive the holy baptism, and be born again in water and spirit to eternal life'. After practicing obstetrics for over 30 years, the author questions the right to risk the life of the mother for the sake of this uncertain creature. Those who refuse to touch the child in severely neglected cases commit manslaughter, and it is 'to God and humanity justifiable' to sacrifice the doomed child in time to save the mother. Necessity knows no law, and God, who 'knows the thoughts of our hearts, he sees to the good intention and the will, but not to the act. Psal. 119:23-24'.[44]

A perilous and fragile condition

This chapter has used close reading of observations of obstetric emergencies to illuminate concepts of fetal and infant viability in the context of late-seventeenth- and early-eighteenth-century Sweden. Highlighting practices

42 Ibid., pp. 78-79.
43 Ibid., pp. 73-75.
44 Ibid., p. 80.

of examination and intervention, it has emphasized the liminal status of perinatal bodies resulting from the ambiguous signs of vitality and decay observed and described by birth practitioners: signs that often reinforced notions of vulnerability, conditionality and passivity.

If exceptional bodies functioned as 'ways to understand and order the world', as suggested in the introduction to this volume, it may be argued that by blending life and death, the liminal and indistinct corporeality of fetuses and infants in early modern birth discourses mediated experiences of, and belief in, the fundamental instability of human existence in a fallen world.

The unborn infant in the case studies published by Johan von Hoorn emerges as a passive bundle of body parts, tightly squeezed, and trapped in a bone cage, unable to move or help itself. It is a creature that seems marginalized, already lost, and abandoned. It appears compressed, lifeless and quiet. The mother, by contrast, is represented in emotionally charged descriptions as vulnerable, courageous and desperate.

The results suggest that the discourse on obstructed birth in the above mentioned manuals was deeply influenced by the determination to intervene manually, and conjured up by haptic experiences conditioned by specific technical limitations that governed birth practices in this context. It was also affected by the importance assigned to the temporary survival necessary to baptism, which demanded complete separation and that the body of the child appear essentially unharmed.

The later manuals testify to a growing resolution on the part of the author-practitioner to promote surgical intervention, by stressing the incidence of intrauterine death. The child and the mother appear in these texts as separate and individual bodies, and their affinity and symbiosis are toned down. This position is partly achieved by recurrent statements that upgrade maternal labour and suffering and declare that the child 'owes its mother gratitude' for giving it life. The biased focus of the case studies, highlighting complications and deviations, and the distinct presence of fetal death lead readers to pursue and complete the more or less unstated argument of the author: that in desperate cases it is morally defensible that the life of the mother has priority over the life of the child.

Nevertheless, counter-images appear – the result of a contradictory discourse. The occasional use of the metaphor of 'imprisonment' for the maternal body suggests how depictions of the double relief of birth may be used to increase compassion for the child. An innocent person, a harmless soul locked up in a cage, a prison-cavity of flesh and bone; entombed alone in the darkness. Ultimately, the power to release this unnaturally positioned unborn infant unharmed was still beyond the horizon, and resided in the hands of God.

The perinatal child in late-seventeenth- and early-eighteenth-century Swedish obstetric emergency discourses remains an elusive creature, because of its general vulnerability, the amount of fetal wastage from which it emerges, and the fluid and indistinct signs with which it manifested itself. Yet the tentative hands of the practitioner, tracing its tangible and unruly contour as it forces the passage, make it visible and present.

Works Cited

Primary Sources

Guillemeau, Jacques, *Child-Birth; or, The Happy Delivery of Women: Wherein Is Set Downe Government of Women* [...] (London, 1635).

Reglemente och Förordning, för Jorde-Gummorne uti Stockholm. Uppå Höga Öfwerhetens Befalning och Approbation Af Kongl. Collegio Medico uthgifwen, Den 29 Aprilis Åhr 1711 (Stockholm, 1736).

Von Hoorn, Johan, *De partu praeternaturali* (Leiden, 1690).

Von Hoorn, Johan, *Den Swenska Wäl-öfwade Jord-Gumman Hwilken Grundeligen underwijser huru med en Hafwande handlas / en Wåndande hielpas / en Barna-Qwinna handteras / och det nyfödda Barnet skiötas skal* [...] (Stockholm, 1697).

Von Hoorn, Johan, *Anatomes publicae* [...] *mirabilia omnipotentis circa generationem humanam* (Stockholm, 1708).

Von Hoorn, Johan, *The Twenne Gudfruchtige / I sitt Kall trogne / och therföre Af Gudi wäl belönte Jordegummor SIPHRA och PUA. Hwilka / Uthi enfaldiga Frågor och Swar En lärgirig Barnmorska troligen underwisa* [...] (Stockholm, 1715).

Von Hoorn, Johan, *Bref til den Edle och Höglärde Doctorn och Anatomiæ Professorn Herr Magnus Bromell Hwaruthi Grundeligen och noga undersökes: Huru wijda man utaf Lungans siunckande eller flytande i watnet, kan med säkerhet döma och sluta: Det Barnet, hwar af Lungan tages, är dödt födt, eller lefwandes i dagsliuset kommit* (Stockholm, 1718).

Von Hoorn, Johan, *The Twenne Gudfruchtige / I sitt Kall trogne / Och therföre Af Gudi wäl belönte Jordegummor SIPHRA och PUA* [...] *Wid denna Andra Uplägningen på många ställen förbättrat; Och med Tolff Historiske Anmärckningar: Samt theras Lärdomar / förökat* [...] (Stockholm, 1719).

Von Hoorn, Johan, *Then Swenska Wälöfwade Jorde-Gummans Andra Deel* [...] (Stockholm, 1723).

Von Hoorn, Johan, *Die Zwo um ihrer Gottesfurcht und Treue willen von GOTT wohl belohnthe Weh-Mütter Siphra und Pua. Welche in Frag und Antwort treulich unterwiesen* [...] (Stockholm, 1726).

Secondary Sources

Bates, Brian, and Allison Newman Turner, 'Imagery and Symbolism in the Birth Practices of Traditional Cultures', in *The Manner Born: Birth Rites in Cross-Cultural Perspective*, ed. Lauren Dundes (Walnut Creek: Altamira Press, 2003), pp. 87-97.

Churchill, Wendy D., *Female Patients in Early Modern Britain: Gender, Diagnosis, and Treatment* (Farnham: Ashgate, 2012).

Cressy, David, *Birth, Marriage, and Death: Ritual, Religion, and the Life-Cycle in Tudor and Stuart England* (Oxford: Oxford University Press, 1997).

Dintler, Åke, *Lars Roberg: Akademiska sjukhusets grundare*, 2nd ed. (Uppsala: Akademiska sjukhuset, 1959).

Djurberg, Vilhelm, *Läkaren Johan von Hoorn: Förlossningskonstens grundläggare i Sverige*, Lychnosbibliotek 4 (Uppsala: Lärdomshistoriska samfundet, 1942).

Douglas, Mary, *Purity and Danger: An Analysis of Concepts of Pollution and Taboo* (London: Routledge, 1966).

Duden, Barbara, *The Woman beneath the Skin: A Doctor's Patients in Eighteenth-Century Germany*, trans. Thomas Dunlap (Cambridge, MA: Harvard University Press, 1991).

Eccles, Audrey, *Obstetrics and Gynaecology in Tudor and Stuart England* (London: Croom Helm, 1982).

Foucault, Michel, *Abnormal: Lectures at the Collège de France, 1974-1975*, ed. Valerio Marchetti and Antonella Salomoni; English series editor, Arnold I. Davidson; trans. Graham Burchell (London: Verso, 2003).

Gélis, Jacques, *History of Childbirth: Fertility, Pregnancy and Childbirth in Early Modern Europe* (Boston: Northeastern University Press, 1991).

Gélis, Jacques, *Les enfants des limbes: Mort-néz et parents dans Europe chretienne* (Paris: Louis Audibert, 2006).

Grell, Ole Peter, 'The Protestant Imperative of Christian Care and Neighbourly Love', in *Health Care and Poor Relief in Protestant Europe 1500-1700*, ed. Andrew Cunningham and Ole Peter Grell (London: Routledge, 1997), pp. 42-63.

Imhof, Arthur E., *Lost Worlds: How Our European Ancestors Coped with Everyday Life and Why Life Is So Hard Today*, trans. Thomas Robisheaux (Charlottesville: University Press of Virginia, 1996).

Keller, Eve, 'The Subject of Touch: Medical Authority in Early Modern Midwifery', in *Sensible Flesh: On Touch in Early Modern Culture*, ed. Elizabeth D. Harvey (Philadelphia: University of Pennsylvania Press, 2003), pp. 62-80.

Laurentius Petris Kyrkoordning av år 1571; utgiven av Samfundet Pro Fide et Christianismo, ed. Emil Färnström (Stockholm: Diakonistyrelsen, 1932).

Marland, Hilary, *Mother and Child Were Saved: The Memoirs (1693-1740) of the Frisian Midwife Catharina Schrader* (Amsterdam: Rodopi, 1987).

McTavish, Lianne, *Childbirth and the Display of Authority in Early Modern France* (Burlington: Ashgate, 2005).
Paulsson Holmberg, Tove, *Onaturlig födelse: Johan von Hoorn och det obstetriska dilemmat 1680-1730* (Lund: Lund University, 2017).
Schwartz, Louis, *Milton and Maternal Mortality* (Cambridge: Cambridge University Press, 2009).
Wilson, Adrian, *The Making of Man-Midwifery: Childbirth in England, 1660-1770* (Cambridge, MA: Harvard University Press, 1995).
Woods, Robert, *Death before Birth: Fetal Health and Mortality in Historical Perspective* (Oxford: Oxford University Press, 2009).

About the Author

Tove Paulsson Holmberg is a post doc researcher in History of Ideas and Sciences, Lund University. Her PhD thesis (2017) examined late-seventeenth- and early-eighteenth-century Swedish midwifery manuals, with a particular focus on obstetric intervention and the development and mediation of epistemic authority.

Afterword

Kathleen Long

Abstract

In the early modern world, exceptional bodies are linked to knowledge, not as the production of knowledge of the self through the scrutiny of those who have been 'othered', but as a means of inducing self-scrutiny and awareness of the limitations of human understanding. Exceptional beings and phenomena entice us to consider the world beyond that which is familiar to us and raise questions concerning our knowledge systems based on notions of what is natural or, in our modern era, normal. Rather than reacting with horror, disgust or pity, we can learn to respect the variety, mobility and resilience of the natural world in our contemplation of that which we see as exceptional.

Keywords: epistemology, eugenics, monstrous, natural philosophy, natural variation, normal

What do we mean by the phrase 'exceptional bodies'? While Foucault claims that '[t]he monster is by definition the exception',[1] exceptional bodies are not necessarily monstrous. An exception is something which is set beyond the limits of the law, set outside of a particular group of things, cut out or eliminated, excluded.[2] These ideas concerning the exception circulated in

1 Foucault, *Abnormal*, p. 58. Foucault does point out earlier that the monster is an extreme among exceptions: 'The monster is the limit, both the point at which law is overturned and the exception that is found in extreme cases' (p. 56).

2 Some examples from Jean Nicot's *Thrésor de la langue françoyse tant ancienne que moderne* (1606) include: '*Tout sans rien excepter, Universus*' (Everything without exception, Universal); '*Excepté nous, Praeter nos*' (Except for us, Beyond us); '*Excepté toy seul, Extra te unum*' (Except for you alone, Outside of you alone); '*Qui est excepté et mis à part, Exceptitius*' (Which is excepted, and set aside, Excluded). These examples can be found at the ARTFL site, *Dictionnaires d'autrefois*, https://artflsrv03.uchicago.edu/philologic4/publicdicos/query?report=bibliography&head=ex cepter (accessed 3 June 2020).

Bondestam, M. (ed.), *Exceptional Bodies in Early Modern Culture: Concepts of Monstrosity before the Advent of the Normal*. Taylor & Francis Group, 2020
DOI 10.5117/9789463721745_AFTER

the realm of the judicial until the late nineteenth century, and policed the boundaries of the law, restricting its scope. In this sense, then, exceptions are not monstrous, unnatural or even necessarily rare, although their existence often evokes these concepts. Nor are they ordinary, for they would be incorporated into the law if they were. The three-legged dove of this volume's introduction does not have an exceptional body, for such a body has become so common as to be ordinary, at least according to Carl Linnaeus.

Somehow, when we are thinking about bodies that perturb us or at least disrupt our understanding of the world, we fall back on rules, mostly of our making, that include or exclude them, organizing them into categories or set them aside as uncategorizable. We have made rules to organize an unruly world, from language, to behaviour, to bodies and other natural phenomena. And over time, many of the concepts driving these rules have come to be associated with exceptional or even monstrous bodies. Before *normal* was used to designate an ordinary or regular body,[3] the word *anormal* was used in French to designate irregular verbs and irregular behaviour, as early as the thirteenth century.[4] The term *normal* comes into usage in the fifteenth century, in the work of Charles d'Orléans.[5] Thus, the concept of the irregular as abnormal precedes that of the regular as normal. Medieval and early modern rules or laws seem to be predicated on the concept of the abnormal or exceptional, rather than that of the normal or ordinary.

But from Roman times, the normal was associated with nature and with the body, as Cicero makes clear in his treatise on sceptical philosophy, the *Academica*: 'that the source of all things good is in the body – this is nature's canon [*normam*] and rule and injunction'.[6] This body is variable and inconstant – or can be seen that way, as it adjusts to changing environments and situations.

In early modern times, this inconstancy or irregularity, when manifested in the body, was associated with the imperfect nature of human knowledge. We seek, and have sought since ancient times, mastery of our environment and ourselves by means of the knowledge systems we elaborate. But these systems are limited in their scope, just as our understanding of the world

3 'État ordinaire et régulier', in *Le Dictionnaire de l'Académie française*.

4 '*Conjugacions anormales, Qui à decliner sont moult males*', from the *Bataille des 7 arts*, and '*Et conferment leurs euvres males / Par exceptions anormales*', Jean de Meun, *Le Roman de la rose*, 19848, cited in the *Dictionnaire de la langue française*.

5 'Normal, ale', in *Le Dictionnaire de l'Académie française*.

6 '*fontem omnium bonorum in corpore esse, hanc normam, hanc regulam, hanc praescriptionem esse naturae*', Cicero, *Academica*, 2.46.140, pp. 648-649.

around us is necessarily limited. And so, Michel de Montaigne can say of the bodies his contemporaries called monstrous:

> What we call monsters are not so to God, who sees in the immensity of his work the infinity of forms that he has comprised in it; and it is for us to believe that this figure that astonishes us is related and linked to some other figure of the same kind unknown to man.[7]

That which we deem monstrous or exceptional is only so in relation to the laws we ourselves make. Thus, we place these bodies outside of the limits of our law, but they also stand outside of our law gazing in, as it were, and force us to reconsider the limitations of the rules we impose so as to give (human) order to our world.

All of the bodies in this volume are seen in relation to this human order of things, and all of them relate to this order in a disorderly way, underscoring its contingency and its own fleeting, inconstant, nature. The *moresca*, a dance form suggesting foreign bodies and disorderly movement, is recuperated by Girolamo Mercuriale as a method of training the body and maintaining its health and orderly functioning. This is achieved through control of bodily movements with the goal of moderating the body and mind, as Maria Kavvadia demonstrates. In this case, a practice at first seen as outside of the realm of rules and proper order is reframed as contributing to corporeal and social order, and thus made unexceptional.

The placement of a monstrous Medusa figure, and the mobile image it resides in, on an early modern fugitive sheet in Johann Remmelin's *Catoptrum microcosmicum*, complicates the negative view of female anatomy by evoking its generative nature, as Rosemary Moore suggests. This figure, its placement, and the images that surround it, encourage us to observe and interpret it more carefully, considering the multiple meanings engendered by the different possible juxtapositions.

Pablo García Piñar analyses how Juan Ruiz de Alarcón's literary achievements form a critique of a bureaucratic system based on promotion of candidates with what we would now call normative bodily attributes. Ruiz de Alarcón contrasts physical deformity and intellectual ability in his plays, raising the question of the viability of these standards. His own body is multiply exceptional, excluded from the governing hierarchy because of its visibly different nature. But he presents his exceptional mind as the

7 Montaigne, *Essays*, bk II, chap. 30, p. 539.

counterweight to this body, seeking to and succeeding in reintegrating himself into the domain of the law.

Cécile Tresfels reveals how Marguerite de Valois's body is deformed in propagandistic political discourses as a critique of her sexuality, which does not conform to social guidelines of the time concerning women's behaviour. This critique reflects both the strict regulation of women's sexuality and her relative independence from these limitations. The rhetoric of this propaganda is itself exceptional, even to the point of the monstrous, in its grotesque representation of Marguerite's body and her sexuality. Parker Cotton considers the use of the hermaphrodite in opening up theological and philosophical questions concerning the nature of the human, calling into question dogmatic understandings of the nature of sin and its impact on humanity in Pierre Bayle's *Dictionnaire historique et critique*. In both of these instances, we see the pressure of the law, of rules and codes, on the exceptional body (or the body supposed to be exceptional). But we also see the resistance that the body might offer to such pressure, opening up new possibilities for contemplating the world around us.

For all of these exceptional bodies are presented as such in relation to human laws, whether represented as natural, theological or social, but they also stand outside of those laws, evoking critiques of these systems or suggesting alternative ways of understanding the world. The effect of these bodies is a revelation of things beyond the current human forms of knowledge, but also as a spur to continue to seek new knowledge. The surprising, awe-inspiring and unexpected capture our attention and push at the limits of our knowledge, causing us to seek to comprehend, rather than resting on what we think we already know. This is the lesson of the prodigies recorded by Johannes Schefferus and analysed by Maja Bondestam. The fisherman's son embodies seemingly contradictory categories (much as the hermaphrodites in Cotton's chapter embody a range of theological and philosophical antinomies): adult/infant, upper/lower, human/animal. In the case of the piglet born with a human-like head, the monster of Lillebered, Schefferus's multiple but still uncertain explanations leave it to the reader to seek an answer; the exceptional bodies and objects he presents to us cause wonder and curiosity that in turn open up further inquiry.

Nowhere is the crucial nature of this search for knowledge – not fixed, dogmatic knowledge, but knowledge that is constantly adapting itself to new information, recalibrating what fits within our 'laws' – more evident than in childbirth, where decisions concerning the status of the infant can be a matter of life and death, as Tove Paulsson Holmberg makes clear. The perinatal infant in the early modern period is an exceptional body in a very different way from the others considered in this volume, embodying the uncertain line between life and death, and evoking the difficulties with trying to interpret that distinction in a body that remained largely invisible to those attempting to deliver it. In no other domain were the limitations of human understanding of the body more painfully evident. In these cases, every body delivered is exceptional, every decision made anew on the basis of shifting circumstances and observations both clear and doubtful.

For whatever reason, we seem to long for a world of certainty, where our knowledge might encompass all of existence, and where everything remains stable and unchanging over time. Perhaps this is why Aristotle imagined perfection residing in bodies resembling that of an ideal type, the father, without variation, and deemed monstrous anything that departed from that type.[8] In this regard, his ideas approach our modern concept of the norm, but without the statistical supports that we have developed to justify this narrow view of humanity and of nature. While Cicero saw exceptional bodies, the monstrous, as prodigies, that is, possible signs of divine will,[9] he also expressed scepticism concerning that belief. Augustine saw natural variation as a sign of the extent of God's power, and our understanding of unusual bodies as monstrous as a sign of the limitations of human knowledge.[10] Like Cicero, Augustine was sceptical about the possibility of reading these bodies with any certainty.[11]

'The exception proves the rule', as the saying goes, but what if the exception were the rule? Montaigne speculates on this possibility in his essay, 'Of Experience', suggesting that '[r]esemblance does not make things so much alike as difference makes them unlike. Nature has committed herself to make nothing separate that was not different.'[12] Most of his essay is a critique of laws intended to put in order an infinite variety of human actions and of knowledge systems elaborated to regularize the natural world. For Montaigne, if the exception *is* the rule, we are constrained to accept our knowledge as contingent, mobile and uncertain, not so that we reject knowledge, but so that we might seek continually to understand the world better. This is the lesson of Schefferus's prodigies as well; that knowledge

8 Long, 'From Monstrosity', pp. 39-40.

9 Davies, *Renaissance Ethnography*, p. 30. For Cicero's scepticism, see his *De divinatione*, bk 2, chaps 31-33, pp. 405-407.

10 Augustine, *City of God*, bk 16, chap. 8, p. 708.

11 Ibid., bk 21, chap. 8, pp. 1063-1064. After a discussion of the meaning of monsters, signs, portents and prodigies, he concludes: 'Let those who divine by such means see for themselves how often they draw false conclusions from them.'

12 Montaigne, *Essays*, bk III, chap. 13, p. 815.

must constantly be revised, improved, expanded to encompass that which we do not yet understand, to include that which has been excluded from the scope of our epistemological systems.

In the modern era, a rigid version of the Aristotelian ideal type, the male Greek aristocrat, was adopted by natural philosophers, anatomists and teratologists who saw evolution as a movement towards a fixed goal, the perfection of various species. There was a perceived urgency to restore order to the natural world, by imposing laws, constructed by man but perceived as natural, on all living beings. This narrow view of evolution, towards an ideal form, was espoused by the proponents of eugenics who sought to eliminate exceptional bodies and thus represented them in a negative light. Eugenicist practices were closely linked to modern breeding practices for animals, and so humans shaped nature according to concepts they had formed in their minds, striving for an idealized conformity that eliminated variation perceived as unnecessary, unaesthetic or useless. These practices were linked to a utilitarian understanding of nature, one that saw the natural world as simply resources for human use and profit, rather than something of value in its own right.[13]

Exceptional bodies decentre the human as well as the normal from our understanding of the world. Georges Canguilhem, like Montaigne, saw variation as natural, affirming that adaptation to particular environments and circumstances would always push the limits of the normal, as well as revealing these limits: 'To the extent that living beings diverge from the specific type, are they abnormal in that they endanger the specific form or are the inventors on the road to new forms?'[14] His work owes a great deal to the Augustinian tradition and its use of exceptional bodies to mark the limits of human knowledge, but also to Montaigne, who used them as incitements to continued questioning of knowledge systems and of the world.

While modern notions of the normal and abnormal are linked to classical, medieval and early modern notions of the monstrous,[15] and the modern natural and medical philosophers Canguilhem cites provide direct links to these earlier concepts,[16] the complexity of early modern discussions of exceptional bodies demonstrates significant differences from modern versions. Aristotelian, Augustinian and Ciceronian traditions coexist in both confrontation and dialogue with each other, complicating any simple view

13 Black, *War against the Weak*, pp. 9-19.
14 Canguilhem, 'A Critical Examination of Certain Concepts', *The Normal*, p. 141.
15 For this link, see Bearden, 'Before Normal'.
16 Long, 'From Monstrosity', pp. 52-58.

of the role of the extraordinary body. The revival of sceptical philosophy becomes entangled in the work of Montaigne with corporeal variation. This connection reveals the centrality of the body to our perceptions, which shape our understanding of the world, thus rendering such knowledge potentially infinitely variable.

So perhaps 'the exception proves the rule', not only in that it tests it or establishes it, but also in that it is the rule because natural variation is fundamental to life itself. Montaigne summarizes this idea in his well-known essay, 'Of Experience': 'Nature has committed herself to make nothing separate that was not different.'[17] Recently, this notion of natural variation has been echoed by scholars writing on the posthuman; Patricia MacCormack adeptly joins postmodern theory with premodern material in her essay on 'Posthuman Teratology', asserting that 'we are all, and must be monsters because nothing is ever like another thing, nor like itself from one moment to the next'.[18] As the studies in this volume suggest, awareness of this fact seems most clear in our reactions to bodies we see as exceptional. We seek to exclude the bodies that resist our urge to impose order or we seek to comprehend them, either by making them fit into the systems we have created or by expanding the scope of these systems. In this choice lies the future of our world.

Works Cited

Augustine, *The City of God against the Pagans*, ed. R.W. Dyson (Cambridge: Cambridge University Press, 1998).

Bearden, Elizabeth B., 'Before Normal, There Was Natural: John Bulwer, Disability, and Natural Signing in Early Modern England and Beyond', *PMLA* 132, no. 1 (2017), pp. 33-50.

17 Montaigne, *Essays*, bk III, chap. 13, p. 815. This essay also presents his critique of knowledge as the organization of the natural and the social worlds, comparing the work of legal and medical scholars to that of children trying to shape mercury: 'The more they press it and knead it and try to constrain it to their will, the more they provoke the independence of this spirited metal; it escapes their skill and keeps dividing and scattering in little particles beyond all reckoning' (p. 816).

18 MacCormack, 'Posthuman Teratology', p. 294. Her Heraclitean take on the inherent mobility of form and identity is reminiscent of Montaigne's portrayal of the self as monstrous: 'I have seen no more evident monstrosity and miracle in the world than myself. We become habituated to anything strange by use and time; but the more I frequent myself and know myself, the more my deformity astonishes me, and the less I understand myself.' Montaigne, *Essays*, bk III, chap. 11, p. 787. His notion of himself as variable seems related to Heraclitus's idea that 'never had a man entered the same river twice' (bk II, chap. 12, p. 455), that is, that we are constantly changing and therefore never the same from 'one moment to the next'.

Black, Edwin, *War against the Weak: Eugenics and America's Campaign to Create a Master Race* (Washington, DC: Dialog Press, 2003).

Canguilhem, Georges, *The Normal and the Pathological*, with an introduction by Michel Foucault, trans. Carolyn R. Fawcett in collaboration with Robert S. Cohen (New York: Zone Books, 1989).

Cicero, Marcus Tullius, *De natura deorum, Academica*, trans. H. Rackham (Cambridge, MA: Harvard University Press, Loeb Classical Library, 1979).

Cicero, Marcus Tullius, *De senectute, De amicitia, and De divinatione*, trans. William Armistead (Cambridge, MA: Harvard University Press, Loeb Classical Library, 2001).

Davies, Surekha, *Renaissance Ethnography and the Invention of the Human: New Worlds, Maps, and Monsters* (Cambridge: Cambridge University Press, 2016).

Dictionnaire de la langue française (Littré, 1873). https://artflsrv03.uchicago.edu/philologic4/publicdicos/query?report=bibliography&head=anormal (accessed 3 June 2020).

Le Dictionnaire de l'Académie française (1835). https://artflsrv03.uchicago.edu/philologic4/publicdicos/query?report=bibliography&head=normal (accessed 3 June 2020).

Long, Kathleen P., 'From Monstrosity to Postnormality: Montaigne, Canguilhem, Foucault', in *Monstrosity, Disability, and the Posthuman in the Medieval and Early Modern World*, ed. Richard H. Godden and Asa Simon Mittman (New York: Palgrave Macmillan, 2019), pp. 35-61.

MacCormack, Patricia, 'Posthuman Teratology', *The Ashgate Research Companion to Monsters and the Monstrous*, ed. Asa Simon Mittman with Peter J. Dendle (Farnham: Ashgate, 2012), pp. 293-310.

Mittman, Asa Simon, 'Introduction: The Impact of Monsters and Monster Studies', in *The Ashgate Research Companion to Monsters and the Monstrous*, ed. Asa Simon Mittman with Peter J. Dendle (Farnham: Ashgate, 2012), pp. 1-14.

Montaigne, Michel de, *Essays*, trans. Donald Frame (Stanford: Stanford University Press, 1958).

About the Author

Kathleen Long is Professor of French in the Department of Romance Studies at Cornell University, author of *Another Reality: Metamorphosis and the Imagination in the Poetry of Ovid, Petrarch, and Ronsard* and *Hermaphrodites in Renaissance Europe*. Her research focuses on gender, religious violence, and disability in early modern France.

Index

For Product Safety Concerns and Information please contact our EU representative GPSR@taylorandfrancis.com
Taylor & Francis Verlag GmbH, Kaufingerstraße 24, 80331 München, Germany

www.ingramcontent.com/pod-product-compliance
Ingram Content Group UK Ltd.
Pitfield, Milton Keynes, MK11 3LW, UK
UKHW021720240926
475702UK00029BA/1671
* 9 7 8 1 0 4 1 1 7 9 0 2 3 *